Acknowledge...

In particular, I would like to thank *Schering ... Care Ltd* & *Condomania Ltd* for supporting publication of *SEXplained 2... For Young People*.

I would like to thank my editor, Penny **Hopkinson** – whose scalpel was mightier than the pen and whose encouragement got me through, and the **Anderson** family for their support.

I would also like to thank:
Faith **Bent**
Phil and Andrea **Costello**
Fergus **Dalgarno**, LLB, Dip PG, Barrister
Leo **Downer** – Director of Brixton Drug Project; author *Crack* – A Worker and Carer's Guide
Julie **Downer**
Chiekezie **Emeribe**
Dr Rimah **El-Borai** – MB BCh, MRCS, LMSSA(Lon) – Instructing Doctor in Family Planning/GP lecturer
Aisha **Ginn**
Peter **Hamilton** – Social Worker
Simon **Ingman**
Michele **Inniss**
Andrew, Wendy and Gemma **Knox** – for asking so many questions as they grew up!
Mr Ali **Kubba** – Consultant Community Gynecologist – for comments on the contraception section
Carol **Lord** – Police Officer, London
Sarah **Moore**, Robbie **Gee** and Eddie **Nestor** – GeeStor Productions Ltd
Denis **O'Brien** – Head of Year – Bishop Thomas Grant School, London
Karin **O'Sullivan** – Family Planning Nurse and Sex Educator
Gary **Pankhurst** – Police Officer, Child Protection Team, London
Lee **Parker** – Youth Worker, south London
Zac **Philipps** – Year Director 10 & 11, Archbishop Tenison's School, London
Sylvia **Rawsthorn** - Health Visitor and Family Planning Nurse – my cartoonist
Miss Christine **Robinso**n – MB BChir, MA, MFFP, MRCOG – Consultant Community Gynaecologist
Dr Eve **Rosser** – Consultant Paediatrician, Director of Child Health, south London
Gill **Sampson**
Dr Fada **Shinewi** – MBChB, MFFP – Consultant in Family Planning
Sheena **Sukumaran** – Brand Manager, Condomania Ltd, UK
TEEMS (Trans European Event Medical Security) – for comments on the personal safety section
Lloyd **Thames**
Michael **van Straten** – Alternative Health Consultant, TV & radio presenter
Alan **Wood** – Male Sexual Health Specialist and School Sex Education Co-ordinator
Francisca, Antoinette and Christopher **William**

Finally, I would like to thank Christine **Carleton**, Steph **Gillings**, Margaret **Norris**, Louise **Pollard**, Jane **Schofield**, Kate **Sweny**, and the other Doctors, Nurses and clerical staff with whom I work in the field of reproductive health.

Special thanks go to my mother, **Margaret**, for her eternal love, support, patience and care.

Helen Knox

SEXplained...® © 1999 Helen Knox

About the Author

Helen Knox trained as a **Registered Nurse** at the **Westminster Hospital, London**, before working as a Senior Staff Nurse at **St Thomas' Hospital A&E Dept, London** and later as a District Nursing Sister in west London. For the past 12 years, she has worked in the field of contraception and sexual health – and since 1991 as an **Outreach Clinical Nurse Specialist in Contraception and Sexual Health** in south London.

In **1994** she was a finalist in the **Nursing Times/3M National Nursing Awards for Innovation in Nursing and Midwifery** for *exceptional work in expanding the outreach work related to Family Planning and Sexual Health.*

Helen has extensive experience in teaching contraception and sexual health to the public as well as her own profession. She works in Family Planning Clinics and teaches in men's prisons, homeless hostels, drug agencies, probation centres, schools, colleges, civic centres and to sex workers – as well as Schools of Nursing and Universities.
Her teaching style is uniquely open and frank – with no holds barred.

SEXplained... The Uncensored Guide to Sexual Health Helen's highly acclaimed first book, published in 1995, covers all the issues relating to sexually transmitted infection and is also written specifically for the public. In this, her first book in the **SEXplained...®** **series**, she pioneers teaching safer sex from the hepatitis prevention viewpoint, rather than the HIV angle, since it is a bigger threat than AIDS.

Medical photographs are reproduced in colour to illustrate, with chilling effect, some increasingly common infections that reinforce her message – and to stimulate discussion.

Since 1995, Helen has appeared frequently on television, given regular radio interviews and taken part in radio phone-ins. She is also a regular contributor to publications reaching a wide cross-section of target audiences.

In February 1998 she became the 'resident' **Virgin Sexpert**, holding the first live online *Sexual Health Cyber Clinic* for Virgin Net. She also answers individual questions via e-mail from her own
SEXplained...® **Website at http://www.sexplained.com**

In the same year, alongside **Robbie Gee** and **Eddie Nestor**, the UK's leading Black comedy duo she appeared in their show *A Wha Me A Go Win.*

Helen is also a medical advisor to **T.E.E.M.S.** paramedic nightclub security, London.

In 1999, she was nominated for **Writer of the Year** and **Publication of the Year** for **SEXplained...®** **Books** and her **Sexual Health Cyber Clinic** for **Innovation of the Year.**

SEXplained 2...

For Young People

by
Helen Knox
RGN, Dip. DN, FP & Adv FP Cert (A08), FAETC
Outreach Clinical Nurse Specialist
in
Contraception
and Sexual Health

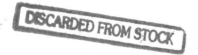

KNOX PUBLISHING
Chiswick, London, UK

First published in 1999.

This book does not seek to condem or condone all or any of the activities or sexual practices described herein. Its intention is to inform only. It is inevitable that a book dealing with sexual health will offend some people. For that, no apology is given. It is only through education that sexual health can improve. This book tries to contribute in a small way to that education.

Signed *H. Knox*

     Helen Knox/Knox Publishing

© Helen Knox 1999

British Library Cataloguing in Publication Data.
A catalogue copy of this book is available from the British Library.

Knox, Helen
    SEXplained 2... For Young People

    ISBN 0-9526224-1-6

Printed in Great Britain by Biddles Ltd.
Medical illustrations by Peter Gardiner.
Cartoon illustrations by Sylvia Rawsthorn.
Cover, page layout, image setting and graphics by Helen Knox, Knox Publishing.
Courtesy condom cartoon illustrations from:
1. The *Getting It On* leaflet, designed in conjunction with FP Sales by Tim Davis MCSD
2. London International Group PLC.

Sex Within the Context of a Loving Relationship

A loving, faithful relationship is built from trust, mutual respect, true friendship and the maturity to work through the tough, as well as the good, times together. As the bond between two individuals deepens, a natural consequence is the desire to start a family and create a secure family unit that will lead to emotional fulfilment.

However, this may take many years to achieve and no one person's journey will be the same. The early years of discovering what you want from a permanent relationship can be exciting, confusing and not without their problems – particularly when what you want doesn't necessarily match the desires of a partner.

This is not the artificial world of movie stars and models, actors and actresses where two people meet, fall in love and live happily ever after within the hour. It is the real world in which real people experience many challenges and face many choices. Making the right choice is so much easier when you have the correct, up to date, relevant and qualified advice about the rewards and risks of sex.

SEXplained 2... For Young People is a book for everyone - regardless of age, race, sexual orientation or disability – to tackle the issues without embarrassment, 'telling it like it is' from the practical viewpoint. It can be used by those working in Sexual Health Education; it can be used by parents to teach their children; young people between the ages of 10 and 24 can read the book for themselves.

SEXplained 2... For Young People brings to life and confronts the many other issues that must be understood in relation to sex and physical relationships. It addresses real questions and real problems from real people from all walks of life – and at every level.

Almost everyone has a little knowledge and a great deal of curiosity about sex. This book does not condone or promote sex below the age of consent. And it won't stop those determined to have underage sex. The more young people know about the many other issues that affect physical relationships, the better able they will be to prevent any problems such as unplanned pregnancy and sexually transmitted infection.

The information in *SEXplained 2... for Young People* will enable its young readers to evaluate both the risks and pleasures of sex before arriving at an informed choice related to their own sexual activity. This will help balance the risks, help people to enjoy their sexuality and develop their sense of responsibility towards each other as well as themselves – without feeling exploited or exploiting others.

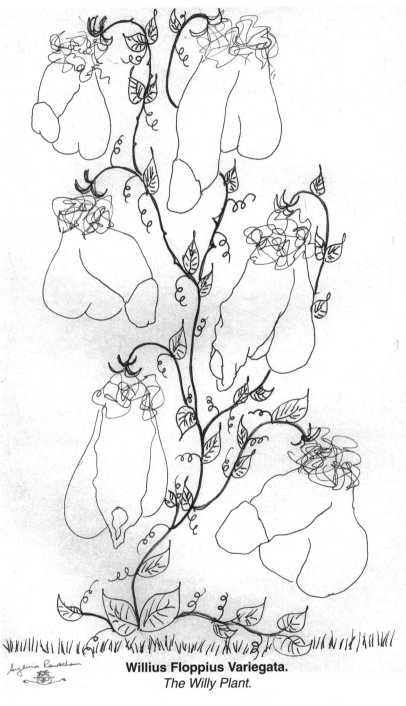

Willius Floppius Variegata.
The Willy Plant.

Puberty and adolescence

- ❖ Puberty is the time when your body starts to change into that of a young man. It happens between the age of about 9 and 18 and lasts for about 4-6 years.
- ❖ Adolescence also occurs around this time, when you mature and change emotionally.
- ❖ In some cultures young men are treated differently by adults when they reach adolescence and there may be a religious celebration eg. the Jewish Barmitzvah ceremony when boys reach the age of 13.

Sperm production

- ❖ During puberty your reproductive organs *(testes)* become active and you produce sperm.
- ❖ Under the influence of chemical and other messages, your brain sends a signal to the tiny tubular areas deep within your testicles, telling them to start producing sperm and the hormone testosterone.
- ❖ Each sperm takes about 76 days to mature. During this time they spend the first 64 days growing into newborn sperm which then move to the epididymis *(still in your testicles)* where they gather, learn to swim and mature over the next 12 days.
- ❖ You can now make a girl pregnant if your sperm comes into contact with her egg.

Quantity of sperm

- ❖ From puberty to old age, if you remain healthy, you'll make thousands of sperm every minute.
- ❖ You'll also have about 3 million sperm in the clear fluid near the tip of your penis each time you get sexually excited *(get an erection)*.
- ❖ An average ejaculation *(come/ cum)* contains about 200-300 million sperm, which is why, in the field of contraception we have a healthy respect for them. It only takes one to lead to pregnancy from so many! A large number of them will be *blanks*, but this still leaves millions of healthy sperm.
- ❖ Sperm may live for up to 7 days inside a female partner if she's at the fertile time of her menstrual cycle and makes fertile mucus for that long.
- ❖ *For further information on the menstrual cycle see page 25-26.*

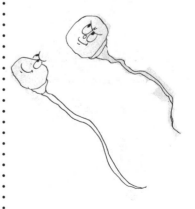

Puberty — male

Testes less than 2.5
cm/1" diameter

Young boy
1 — preadolescent

Testes more than 2.5
cm/1" diameter

Start of puberty
2 — Enlargement of testes; scrotum
enlarges, becomes redder and rougher.
Sparse growth of long hairs at base of penis

Early teens
3 — penis lengthens; more
growth of testes and scrotum.
Darker, thicker, curly hair.

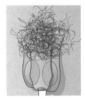

Late teens
4— penis broader ; glans develops; scrotum
darkens.
Hair is adult in type but not as extensive

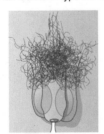

Testes 5-6 cm/2-3$\frac{1}{2}$"
average length

Young adult
5 — adult, hair spreading up towards tummy and to thighs.

Some other changes during puberty

❖ Your voice will start to deepen in tone or *break*.
❖ Hair will start growing on your face, in your pubic area, under your arms, on your chest, arms and legs.
❖ You may develop spots on your face, due to the chemical changes taking place in your body.
❖ The odour *(smell)* of your body may change slightly.
❖ Your penis and testicles will grow in length, width and weight.
❖ You'll grow in height – have a *growth spurt*.
❖ You may have some *wet dreams (ejaculate in your sleep)* occasionally.
❖ You'll gradually become more inquisitive about sex and the mysteries surrounding it.
❖ You'll start to explore your body and learn to masturbate. This won't make you blind, deaf or drive you mad as people used to say in olden days!
❖ You may become interested in fashion, fast cars, music, members of the opposite sex and in the appearance of your body.

Sexuality

❖ You'll probably wonder about your sexuality *(sexual preference)* as you learn to express yourself in the adult world.
❖ As you mature you may become attracted to members of the opposite sex.
❖ You may, however, become attracted to members of your own sex or perhaps both sexes.
❖ *For further information on sexuality see page 118.*

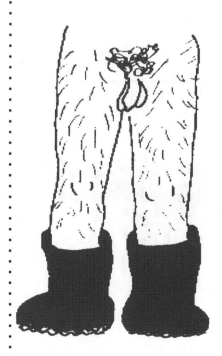

How do boys and men get an erection?

❖ Several things can bring on an erection.

❖ Usually, it's in response to something sexual or exciting. *(Though sometimes it may happen when you're just sitting at the back of a bus, thinking of your maths homework or even a cheese sandwich!)*

❖ Stimulation may be visual, by touch, smell, using your imagination or from memory.

❖ Sometimes, though, an erection happens because of fear.

❖ When sexually stimulated, the muscle at the base of your penis allows blood to flow in. It enlarges, hardens and expands. It then tightens to keep your penis muscles full of blood.

❖ After ejaculation this tight band of muscle relaxes and allows the blood to flow out of your penis again.

❖ You can't pass urine while you have an erection so don't worry that you might pass urine inside your partner during sex — and you may find it difficult to pass urine until your erection goes down — especially early in the morning when you wake up with your early morning erection and full bladder.

A penis cut through to show how an erection occurs

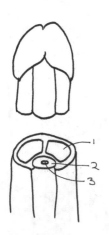

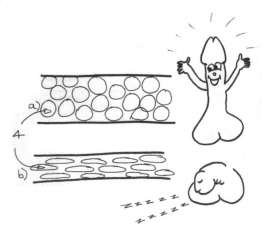

| 1 | Corpus cavernosum | 3 | Urethra (urine passage) |
| 2 | Corpus spongiosum | 4 | Lacunar spaces |

    (a)   filled with blood while erect.
    (b)   collapsed when relaxed (flaccid).

Vital note to all men on pregnancy and sexually transmitted infections

- ❖ Penetration and/or ejaculation are NOT always necessary for a young woman to get pregnant.
- ❖ If your erect unprotected penis comes into contact with a young woman's fertile mucus *(see menstrual cycle on page 23)* sperm can swim into her vagina, up to her uterus, over to her fallopian tubes and she could become pregnant ***without having penetrative sex***!
- ❖ It's important to realise that there are active sperm *(about 3 million)* in the tiny amount of clear fluid, which usually appears at the tip of your penis on erection.
- ❖ To ensure absolutely no risk of pregnancy you must keep an unprotected penis away from female genitalia.
- ❖ If sperm can pass, so can germs, so be extremely careful where you allow your fluids to go, or what you allow them to contact.
- ❖ Even when protection is used, there's still a risk of passing infection both ways if protection fails.
- ❖ *Note: You're at your most virile between the age of 14 and 24 and at your sexual peak, at this time your penis has a mind of its own!*
- ❖ Your penis may not be as choosy as you are! So keep your brain in your head when your erection throbs and remember to protect yourself at all times.

Does it matter that I have a small penis?

- ❖ Size is no barrier to or indication of pleasure.
- ❖ A small penis can receive and give just as much pleasure as a bigger one.
- ❖ Men of all ages, in all countries are obsessed by penis size.
- ❖ Size is irrelevant when it comes to pregnancy or sexual performance.
- ❖ Of course, when it's soft it may appear small, looking down on it as you do from above. Try looking at it sideways in the mirror for a more impressive view!
- ❖ When soft, a small penis can more than double in size by the time it's erect; large penises when soft, don't tend to react so impressively.
- ❖ At times, it might also look larger or smaller – which is also quite usual.
- ❖ Many men don't see other penises erect for comparison! It's perfectly common to have an erection between 5 and 7 inches long.
- ❖ How you measure the length of your penis can add about an inch or two!

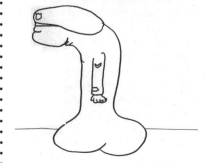

How do I measure the length of my penis?

❖ Measure your penis when you have a good erection. Push it horizontal *(at a right angle to your tummy)* then measure from your hairline to the tip and hey presto, you have its length.

❖ No doubt you could measure from the underside and add an inch or so, with perhaps even more if you measure the back while it's erect instead of horizontal.

❖ There's no reason at all to panic about penis size. It is what it is.

❖ It grows in length, weight and size as you grow up and mature physically.

❖ Some are long, some are short, some are fat and some are thin.

❖ When it's erect, you should feel as proud of it as any other man.

❖ Men often worry about penis size. It's how you use it that really matters, not how much you've got!

I'm worried that my penis is too small for sex and that if someone sees it they'll laugh and not want me any more

❖ Don't worry – you're not alone. You'd be surprised how many men worry about this unnecessarily.

❖ Young men develop at different rates. For example, seeing someone the same age at school with a bigger penis, when you're having a shower after PE, can do untold harm to some young men's egos.

❖ Few heterosexual *(straight)* men get to see another man's penis except if they're watching a pornography film or in the *gents*.

❖ Pornography films sometimes employ trick photography to make a penis look bigger.

❖ A penis that's large when flaccid *(soft)* doesn't usually impress as much as a smaller one does when it erects.

❖ A smaller penis can more than double in size on erection

❖ A larger penis may just increase slightly in length or width. So, you should try not to worry.

How can I make my penis bigger?

❖ Trying to make your penis bigger can cause far more problems than it solves.

❖ Generally you can't enlarge it naturally.

❖ Its size is determined by your genes, which also determine the colour of your eyes, hair etc.

❖ It tends to grow thicker and longer as you mature physically. Your testicles also develop in size and weight.

❖ Some men go to great trouble to try and get surgery or use stretching instruments to lengthen it or have fat injections to make it wider. But many are bitterly disappointed with the expensive lack of results.

❖ Creams, lotions, potions, and surgery are largely a waste of money and just play on your insecurities; they can't guarantee success and often fail to deliver what is eagerly expected.

❖ The psychological damage *(in your mind)* could make the problem far greater and your performance worse than it was before if the result isn't as you hope.

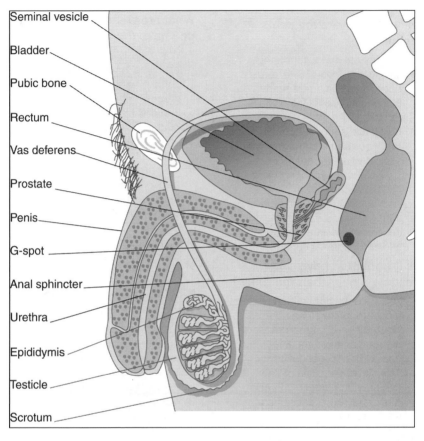

- Seminal vesicle
- Bladder
- Pubic bone
- Rectum
- Vas deferens
- Prostate
- Penis
- G-spot
- Anal sphincter
- Urethra
- Epididymis
- Testicle
- Scrotum

Cross section of male anatomy

- ❖ The average vagina is only 3½" - 4" deep, although it can expand to about twice this, when a penis is inserted slowly and gently, so there's no point in men bragging that they're 12"-14" long! It simply isn't necessary.
- ❖ *Mr. Average* is just fine and preferred, by most partners, long term.
- ❖ *Mr. Huge* is OK for novelty value but can cause discomfort.
- ❖ Believe it or not, it can even lead to couples splitting up.

- ❖ Remember: you should concentrate on how you use what you've got; not how little or how much you have.

Willy Worries

How can I make my penis smaller?

- ❖ In theory to make your penis smaller you *could* have surgery. But it would be a rare man indeed who thinks his penis is too large!
- ❖ If you are seriously concerned that your penis is too big, you should consult your Doctor.
- ❖ Trying to make your penis larger or smaller can lead to more problems, physical and emotional, than you may already have. Just accept what nature's given you and don't worry about size.

Is it normal to have one testicle bigger than the other?

- ❖ Yes, it's quite normal to have one bigger than the other.
- ❖ The left one is often slightly bigger than the right and it usually hangs a bit lower.
- ❖ This clever design is probably so that they don't crash into each other and cause pain when you're running!

What happens to the unused sperm if I don't have sex?

- ❖ After a month or so, the unused sperm degenerate *(break down)* and are absorbed back into your body *(through special areas called sterocilia in the epididymis of your testes)* and are filtered out of your body like any other waste *(eg. in your urine or faeces)*.

What are wet dreams and why do I have them?

- ❖ Wet dreams are when you ejaculate in your sleep due to something sexually arousing in a dream.
- ❖ Wet dreams are also called *nocturnal emissions*.
- ❖ They're perfectly normal and nothing to worry about.
- ❖ Your dream may not have been sexy or about someone you fancy. Wet dreams sometimes happen when they're least expected.
- ❖ Some young men don't have them very often while others have them frequently.

Why do I have an erection when I wake up?

- ❖ It's quite usual to have about 5 erections in your sleep each night, throughout your life.
- ❖ They're more likely to be a left over erection from the last dream you were having before you woke up.
- ❖ These are sometimes nicknamed *piss hards, morning glories* or *dawn horns*.
- ❖ They're not, as is often thought, due to having a full bladder when you wake up and need to *'piss'*.

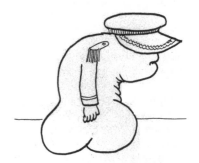

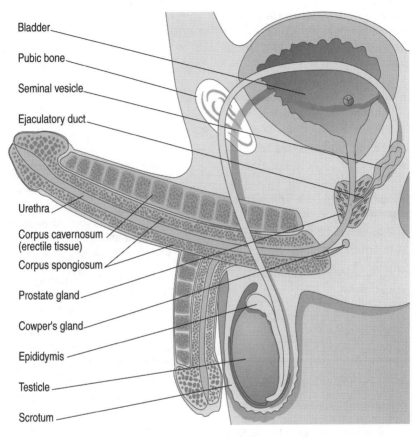

Bladder
Pubic bone
Seminal vesicle
Ejaculatory duct
Urethra
Corpus cavernosum (erectile tissue)
Corpus spongiosum
Prostate gland
Cowper's gland
Epididymis
Testicle
Scrotum

Cross section of male anatomy – showing flaccid and erect penis

Is it normal to have lumps or little bumps on my penis?

❖ You have lots of tiny glands near the tip *(glans)* of your penis, around the coronal sulcus *(crown/helmet)* which may or may not be easily visible as lumps and bumps when you reach puberty.

❖ If you've had them for years and they haven't changed, they're unlikely to be anything to worry about.

❖ If, however, you notice new lumps or bumps and you've had sex in the last few months, it's worth asking a Doctor to check them at a GUM clinic, in case they're genital warts – or another infection.

If I masturbate and stop my ejaculate coming out by squeezing my penis *(or put my finger over its tip or behind my testicles and press hard)* will it do me harm?

❖ In the short term, this is unlikely to do you harm but it's better to ejaculate into a tissue which you can then throw away.

I get a pleasant sensation when I climb frames or ropes in PE at school from rubbing my genital area. Is this an orgasm?

❖ It could well be an orgasm – or a similar sensation.

❖ A young man may get a sensation similar to orgasm with or without ejaculation.

❖ Ejaculation and orgasm are two separate things, yet many people think they're the same. You can have an orgasm without ejaculating and you can ejaculate without having an orgasm.

❖ Most young women reach orgasm through clitoral stimulation. So you're probably getting some form of sexual arousal and pleasure when you rub your genital area against the frame or rope.

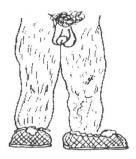

My friends say they go on for ages when they have sex but I ejaculate very quickly. Is this normal?

❖ There's no normal length of time for having sex but this could be called *premature ejaculation*.

❖ It's extremely common when you're very excited at the prospect of having sex, particularly when you're young or with a new sexual partner.

❖ With practice you can have your orgasm and ejaculation as and when you choose.

❖ You can ejaculate without having an orgasm and you can have an orgasm without ejaculating, though they often happen simultaneously *(together)*.

❖ If you are still worried about it refer to the end of this book for further reading about men and sex.

Why do some men get painful erections with their penis bending to one side?

❖ This is a condition more common in middle aged and older men.

❖ It's called Peyronie's disease and is when the muscle on one side of the penis is blocked by little lumps deep inside and it can't fill with blood properly to give a straight erection.

❖ Sometimes sex becomes very difficult and medication or surgery may be recommended.

❖ The reason why it happens to some and not to others is unclear.

How do I put my penis into my partner so we can have sex and does it hurt?

* You need to have a firm erection, not a soft penis.
* A young woman must be turned on enough for sex, making a welcoming fluid, which makes penetration *(entry of your penis into her vagina)* easier and more comfortable.
* If she's not moist you may need to use extra lubrication otherwise penetration may be uncomfortable.
* Gently rub the tip of your penis between the lips *(labia)* of her moist vulva then slowly push your penis inside her vagina.
* Having sex shouldn't hurt either of you.
* *For further information about lubricants see pages 154-5.*

Will my penis be trapped inside my partner when I have sex and how do I get it out again?

* Your penis cannot become trapped because the vagina doesn't trap or 'bite' it.
* So just pull it out gently when you want to withdraw.
* Rarely, some women develop a condition called vaginismus. Their vaginal muscles go into spasm and tighten. It doesn't last long and you can still withdraw your penis easily.

When my penis is inside my partner, will I pass urine?

* No, you can't pass urine while you have an erection.
* A valve at your bladder closes when your penis is erect. This allows semen and sperm to come out through your urethra but it holds your urine back, inside your bladder.

Why do my testicles ache so much when we're just heavy petting?

* During sexual arousal your testicles rise towards your body and swell.
* At orgasm they relax and return to their usual size quite quickly.
* So, if you're just teasing/petting each other for a long time, without ejaculation, they may ache later.
* That doesn't mean you have to have sex to prevent this feeling.
* It'll wear off on its own or after sex – but you can always masturbate to relieve any discomfort. *(It is natural for most men to masturbate. Many are too shy to admit it to their friends or talk about it in company.)*

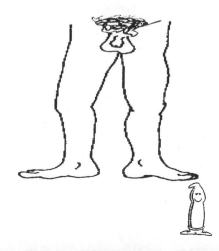

Will my penis be too big to go inside my girlfriend if she's never had sex before?

❖ No, it's unlikely that your penis will be too big. As long as you're gentle, and she's nicely relaxed, aroused and wet, it should slide in easily.

❖ She has to be relaxed otherwise the *welcoming fluid* won't flow to lubricate her vagina.

❖ Her hymen may still be intact if she hasn't used tampons or stretched it during exercise. *(For further information on hymen, see page 42.)*

❖ You should be very gentle, not in a hurry and be ready to stop if she feels pain or changes her mind – even at the last minute.

❖ There's a band of muscle at the entrance to her vagina, which relaxes when she's ready to allow you to enter.

❖ Her vagina has a *dead end* so you don't have to worry about going in too far.

❖ Discuss your decision to have sex carefully though, because once it's lost, she can't retrieve her virginity.

❖ You should also make sure you use adequate protection from pregnancy and/or infection.

❖ She may be at risk of infection if you've had sex before.

❖ Many girls are bullied by peer pressure and made to feel they should have sex by a certain age. There's no upper age limit for having sex, no hurry to start and no right or wrong number of times to *do it*.

❖ *For further information on date rape and Young People, Sex and the Law see pages 121 & 164.*

I can get my penis into my partner but I can't ejaculate. What's wrong and how can I *come*?

❖ Many men worry about not being able to ejaculate inside their partner although they can ejaculate when masturbating.

❖ You need to learn to relax and let go of your worries and your ejaculate.

❖ The reason you hold back may be as simple as being scared of getting your partner pregnant.

❖ Something might have happened to you when you were younger which you subconsciously block out.

❖ There may be other reasons, which you need to explore.

❖ Your GP or Family Planning Clinic Doctor may be able to help you find the reason more easily or refer you to someone else for help.

Does it mean I have sperm if I have erections?

❖ Babies and small boys have erections but don't have sperm.

❖ Sperm start to develop from puberty.

❖ After that, unless a Doctor tells you otherwise, you should assume you have millions of sperm at the tip of your penis every time you have an erection.

❖ There could be enough to cause pregnancy if they get near a young woman's fertile mucus *(even externally)* so be very careful where you put your erect penis!

At what age will I have sperm?

- You start to have sperm soon after you reach puberty.
- This is usually between 10 and 14 years of age.

Should I be able to see sperm in my urine?

- No, sperm are so tiny they're invisible to the naked eye.
- The fluid you ejaculate consists of sperm, semen and prostatic fluid – not all sperm.

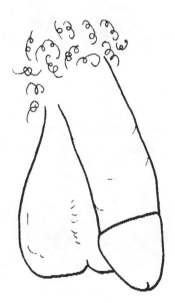

Information about sperm!

- Some people nickname them *tadpoles* because they look similar under a microscope!
- They can swim at about 1/10th of an inch a minute, which is about 6 inches an hour or 0.0001 mph. They come shooting out at an average speed of about 28 miles an hour, along with semen and other alkaline *(non-acid)* fluid in which they're swept along. Without this they'd be killed as soon as they reach the acid of the vagina.
- Some ejaculations may be slower and some faster!
- Sperm get into the cervix after about 90 seconds after ejaculation.
- They can then take only five minutes to reach the fallopian tubes.
- They can live inside a woman for half a day or up to 7 days, depending on the woman's fertile mucus, in which they live, and off which they feed.
- *For information about sperm production, smoking and high blood pressure, see page 32-33.*

If you respect yourself and your partner, you'll want to read Helen's books and pay heed!

Judith Jacob
Actress

Willy Worries

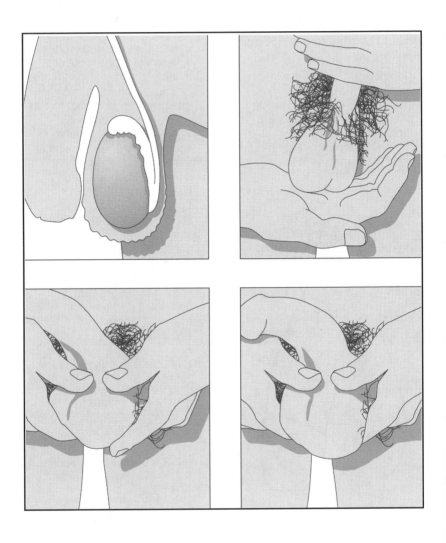

Testicular Self-Examination (TSE)

Testicular Self-Examination (TSE)

A good reason for fiddling with your own or your partner's testicles!

* *All men and boys should be testicle aware — just as ladies are taught to be breast aware.*
* The aim is to catch early signs of cancer of the testicles or other testicular problems.
* Testicular cancer is not a sexually transmitted infection but can affect sexual health and fertility, if it's not treated quickly.
* Men between the ages of 15 and 35 are most commonly affected.
* The incidence of testicular cancer is on the increase. Fortunately it has the highest treatment success rate of all cancers. Don't panic if you notice something unusual.
* Other things can cause swellings or lumps, so it's essential that you let a doctor check you quickly – even if you're embarrassed to ensure the correct diagnosis and treatment.
* The cause of testicular cancer is not proven but the main factors, which may increase your risks, are:

1– age – highest risk 15 to 35 years old.
2– if you had undescended testicles when you were born and needed an operation to bring one or both of them down into your scrotum.
3– infection.
4 – trauma/accident/injury.

How often should I check?

* Check them about once a month.

Where should I check them?

* Checking them in a bath or shower is a good idea, when your scrotum is relaxed and they hang a bit lower.

How do I check them?

* The first time you check them you'll notice various lumps and bumps. Consider these to be your *base line* from which you can notice any changes.
* Rest your testicles in the palm of your hand and note their weight and size.
* You'll probably notice that one testicle is larger than the other and may also hang lower than the other one, which is quite normal.
* Then roll each testicle, in turn, between your thumbs and fingers.
* Feel right round each one and up into your groin behind them.
* You'll notice a spermatic cord behind each testicle *(long, thin, round, semi-hard area)*.
* Look at your testicles in the mirror and notice any visual changes.

SEXplained...® © 1999 Helen Knox

Willy Worries

What else should I look out for?

❖ Look out for a dull ache in your groin or abdomen.
❖ Heaviness in your scrotum.
❖ Occasionally there may be pain in your testicle itself.

I've noticed something

❖ First, check to see if it is on your other testicle, too.
❖ If it is, it's extremely unlikely to be cancer, as it rarely develops on both sides.

Now what do I do?

❖ Make an appointment to see a Doctor – either visit your GP or you can go to a GUM Clinic where the Doctors specialise in dealing with this part of the body and appointments are not always necessary.

What if I've got it?

❖ When it's detected early, simple removal of the affected testicle is usually all that's necessary.
❖ You may be offered special drug or x-ray treatment afterwards.
❖ There's virtually a 100% cure rate when caught early.

I won't look normal any more

❖ Testicular implants (false ones) will probably be discussed with you, so you'll look as you did before.

What about sex?

❖ You'll be able to continue your sex life as before.
❖ The other testicle will continue to produce millions of sperm so your fertility shouldn't be affected.

I've heard of torsion of the testicles, what's that?

❖ Torsion is when a testicle gets twisted in your scrotum and its blood and oxygen supply are cut off.
❖ It's extremely painful and requires medical attention, quickly.
❖ The affected testicle may have to be removed but you still have the other one to make millions of sperm, so your future fertility shouldn't be affected.
❖ As before, you can have a false one implanted to make you look as you did before.

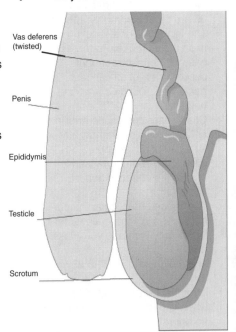

Vas deferens (twisted)

Penis

Epididymis

Testicle

Scrotum

View of testicular torsion

Willy Worries

What's a hydrocele?

❖ Hydrocele is when fluid gathers in your scrotum and it swells up due to a tiny fluid leak from your abdomen to the area surrounding your testicles.

❖ It's common in babies but also common in adult men.

❖ It may or may not be painful depending upon the cause.

❖ It may be due to injury or infection, though it often develops for no known reason.

Depending upon the cause, treatment consists of either

1. Leaving it alone and seeing if it goes away on its own, if it isn't particularly large or painful.
2. Antibiotics if there's an infection.
3. Draining it with a needle *(aspiration)*.
4. Surgical repair if the leak is recurrent, of particular concern or if your scrotum becomes very large and uncomfortable.

View of hydrocele

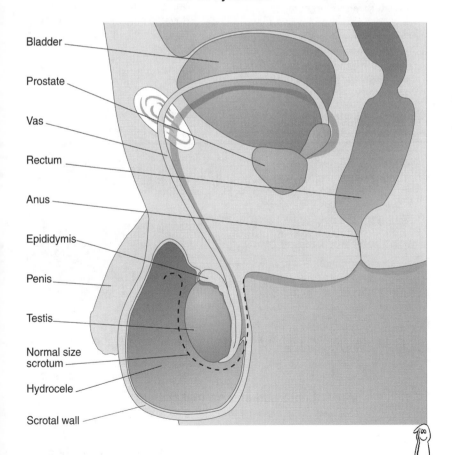

Bladder

Prostate

Vas

Rectum

Anus

Epididymis

Penis

Testis

Normal size scrotum

Hydrocele

Scrotal wall

Willy Worries

What's my prostate?

- ❖ Your prostate is a walnut sized organ or gland, which lies underneath your bladder.
- ❖ It produces a fluid which mixes with semen and sperm during ejaculation.

There are three conditions you should be aware of.

These are related to your prostate and each needs medical attention.

1. Inflammation or infection due to sexually transmitted infections, which *can affect men of all ages.*
2. Benign enlargement *(not cancer)* is very common and affects 1 man in 3 over the *age of 50.*
3. Cancer of the prostate *(malignant)* causes the second highest number of cancer deaths amongst men after lung cancer.

For all three you are likely to notice some or all of the following

- ❖ Altered urination – you may have difficulty or delay when starting to pass urine.
- ❖ Your urine may not flow normally, but may stop and start.
- ❖ You may feel your bladder hasn't emptied properly when you've passed urine.
- ❖ You may have to get up in the night to pass urine, which is not directly related to a *drinking binge* the night before.
- ❖ There's a blood test which can detect if you're more likely to develop cancer of the prostate. Early detection makes treatment easier.

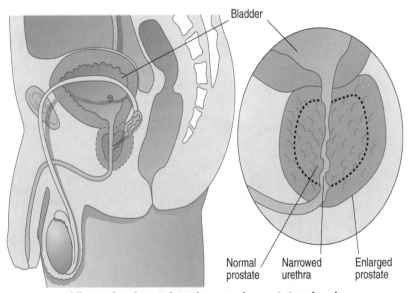

Bladder

Normal prostate / Narrowed urethra / Enlarged prostate

View of enlarged and normal prostate gland
For labels see previous illustration of male anatomy — page 17

Willy Worries

With infection you may notice:

* lower back pain.
* pain on passing urine.
* fever and/or chills.
* general discomfort in your genital area.
* treatment depends upon the cause but consist of antibiotics for infection, surgery or chemotherapy if benign or cancerous *(malignant)* plus additional radiotherapy for cancerous enlargement.

Further genital hygiene

* Good genital hygiene is important to prevent infection.
* If you haven't been circumcised, you should look after your foreskin *(skin fold at tip of penis)*.
* No man is immune from infection but uncircumcised men are at increased risk of contracting sexually transmitted infections.
* A creamy lubricant called smegma, forms underneath it, to keep it moving freely over the tip *(glans)* of your penis.

* Like many other young men, you may know of your smegma by a nickname such as *knob cheese*!
* It's important to wash every day otherwise germs can multiply and your foreskin may become infected, dry and sore, causing it to tighten over the end of your penis *(phimosis)* and become painful.
* You should pull your foreskin back along the shaft of your penis, so that the skin lies flat.
* Wash away the smegma from around the tip area with soap and water before towelling yourself dry again.
* If you're unable to pull your foreskin back to clean underneath it, you may need circumcision.
* Women also make a small amount of smegma around their clitoris, so daily washing is recommended for women, too.
* Women don't suffer from the same tightening as men, so there's no medical reason for female circumcision.
* *For further information on circumcision see page 133.*

View of male genitalia from below

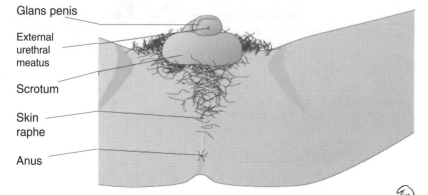

Glans penis

External urethral meatus

Scrotum

Skin raphe

Anus

Puberty — female

Breast development

1 — preadolescent

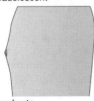

Start of puberty
2 — breast bud — small mound;
areola enlarges

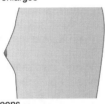

Early teens
3 — further growth; areola and nipple
not separate from breast curve

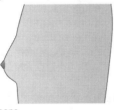

Late teens
4— nipple and areola above curve
of breast

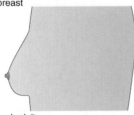

Yound adult
5 — mature: nipple elevated but areola
flattens into breast curve

Pubic hair development

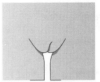

1 — preadolescent

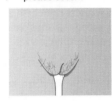

2 — sparse growth of long
hairs on labia

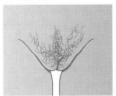

3 — darker, thicker, curly hair
covers junction of pubes

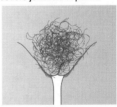

4— adult in type b ut not as extensive

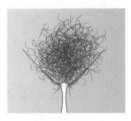

5 — adult in type; spreading up linea alba
and on to medial aspects of the thighs,
especially in males

SEXplained...® © 1999 Helen Knox

What's puberty?

❖ Puberty is the time when your body starts to change from that of a child into a young woman. It happens between the age of about 9 and 16 and lasts for about 3-6 years.

❖ You'll start to release your eggs *(ovulate)* and have periods right through until you're about 50.

❖ Your breasts will start to develop.

❖ You may get spots appearing on your face due to hormonal *(chemical)* changes.

❖ Both your pubic and underarm hair will start to grow.

❖ When you start your periods you'll become a young woman, capable of reproduction. Generally, because of this, your parents or other adults will worry about you and become protective.

What's the difference between puberty and adolescence?

❖ Puberty is the time when you mature physically.

❖ Adolescence is the time when you start to mature emotionally.

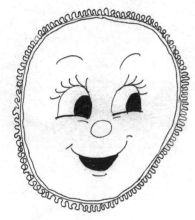

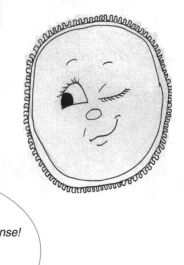

She may be my Auntie but she really does talk a lot of sense!

Gemma Knox
Niece — Aged 17

Egg release

❖ From the start of your periods you will usually release one or two eggs *(ova)* every month.

❖ You were born with your lifetime's supply of eggs in your ovaries.

❖ For this to happen, your brain sends a chemical message in the form of a hormone, FSH *(follicle stimulating hormone),* to your ovaries.

❖ Your ovaries then start to develop an egg for that month and produce oestrogen.

❖ After the egg is released from your ovary, it is wafted along your fallopian tube towards the lining of your womb *(the endometrium)* and your ovary then makes another hormone called progesterone.

View of egg release from ovary

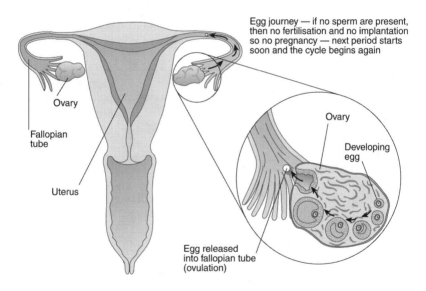

Egg journey — if no sperm are present, then no fertilisation and no implantation so no pregnancy — next period starts soon and the cycle begins again

Ovary

Fallopian tube

Uterus

Ovary

Developing egg

Egg released into fallopian tube (ovulation)

Fertile mucus

❖ The neck of your womb *(cervix)* makes a fertile type of mucus while your egg develops.

❖ You can not get pregnant without fertile mucus present.

❖ Some women make fertile mucus for only a day, while others make it for several days.

❖ It's clear and stretchy, rather like egg white and it's essential for sperm to make their way to your egg.

❖ Sperm can live in it and feed off it for the length of time you make fertile mucus.

❖ After egg release, it changes to infertile or thick mucus which sperm can't get through.

❖ This lasts until you have your next period.

What happens when you have unprotected sex?

❖ At any time, but especially at the fertile time of the month, sperm can travel through the fertile mucus in the neck of your womb *(cervix)*, up through your uterus *(womb)* and into your fallopian tubes where they may meet an egg. They may then join together *(fertilise)*, start to divide and multiply into an embryo.

❖ The embryo spends 3 days travelling back towards the lining of your womb *(endometrium)* before it finds somewhere suitable to implant *(settle)* and start growing into a foetus.

❖ When it implants, a signal is sent from your ovary, telling the lining of your womb to stay in place so you don't have your next period.

❖ It then takes 9 months for the foetus to develop fully into a baby.

❖ You may also be at risk of catching a sexually transmitted infection when you have unprotected sex.

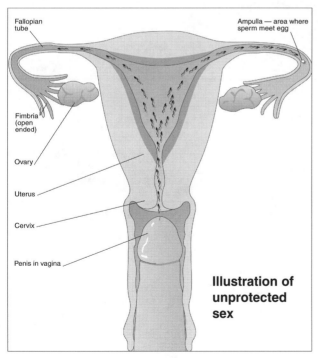

Fallopian tube

Ampulla — area where sperm meet egg

Fimbria (open ended)

Ovary

Uterus

Cervix

Penis in vagina

Illustration of unprotected sex

Ectopic pregnancy

❖ An ectopic pregnancy is where a fertilised egg *(ovum)* and pregnancy develops outside the uterus eg. in the fallopian tube, ovary or abdomen.

❖ The most common area for ectopic pregnancies is in the fallopian tube, when the fertilised egg *(ovum)* gets stuck and settles there, instead of travelling to the lining of your womb to settle.

❖ Ectopic pregnancy could be life-threatening and you would need emergency treatment or surgery to prevent serious illness or even death.

❖ You may have pelvic pain and abnormal vaginal bleeding with ectopic pregnancy.

❖ If worried, you should be checked by your Doctor or visit your local Family Planning Clinic immediately.

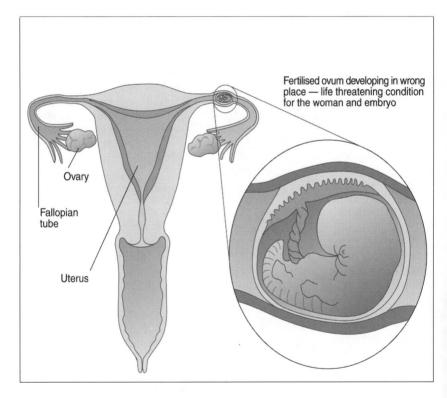

Fertilised ovum developing in wrong place — life threatening condition for the woman and embryo

Ovary

Fallopian tube

Uterus

Ectopic pregnancy

How periods happen

❖ Periods happen because of a series of events throughout your menstrual cycle.

❖ While the egg is being produced in your ovary, the lining of your womb builds a ripe cushion for an ovum *(fertilized egg)* to implant.

❖ If one doesn't implant, it gets a signal from your ovary and the cushion or lining sheds away.

❖ This shedding is what happens when you have your menstrual *(ie. monthly)* period.

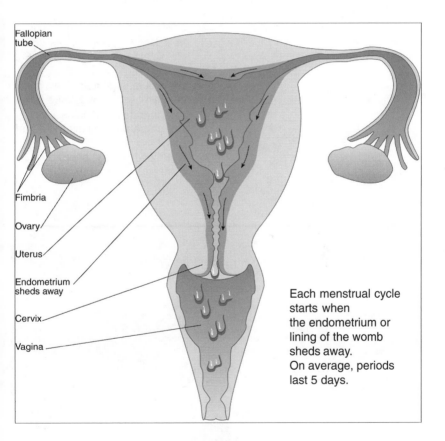

Fallopian tube

Fimbria

Ovary

Uterus

Endometrium sheds away

Cervix

Vagina

Each menstrual cycle starts when the endometrium or lining of the womb sheds away. On average, periods last 5 days.

Lining of the womb shedding

How much blood is lost during a period?

* On average 1-2 tablespoons of blood are lost each month.
* Many people think pints of blood are lost, but this is not true. A little bit of blood can go a long way!
* Some women have heavier periods and may benefit from using hormonl contraception to reduce their blood loss.
* If you are worried about your periods, seek advice from your Doctor or Family Planning Clinic.

How long do periods last and how often do they come?

* Each period will usually last between 3 and 10 days.
* Periods may be irregular for many months while your body adjusts but they usually settle into a pattern of coming between every 21 and 35 days.
* You'll develop your own menstrual pattern and release your egg somewhere between 10 and 16 days before the first day of your *next* period – not always as is often stated, on the 14th day into your cycle.
* Life would be simple if this were the case – there would be fewer unplanned pregnancies. Unfortunately life isn't quite that easy!
* Some people call periods menses, monthlies or *the curse*.

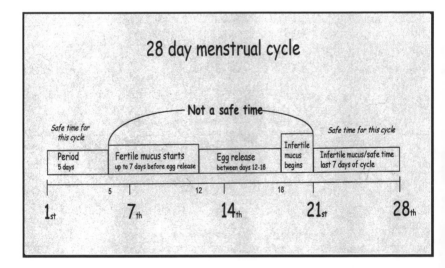

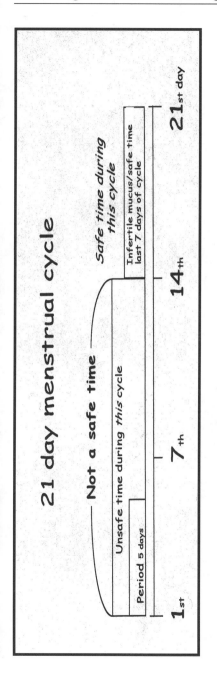

21 day menstrual cycle

— Not a safe time

Safe time during this cycle

Unsafe time during this cycle

Period 5 days

Infertile mucus/safe time last 7 days of cycle

1st   7th   14th   21st day

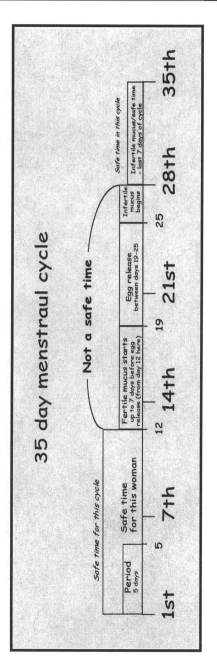

35 day menstraul cycle

Safe time for this cycle

Not a safe time

Safe time in this cycle

Period 5 days

Safe time for this woman

Fertile mucus starts up to 7 days before egg release (from day 12 here)

Egg release between days 19-25

Infertile mucus begins

Infertile mucus/safe time – last 7 days of cycle

1st   5   7th   12   14th   19   21st   25   28th   35th

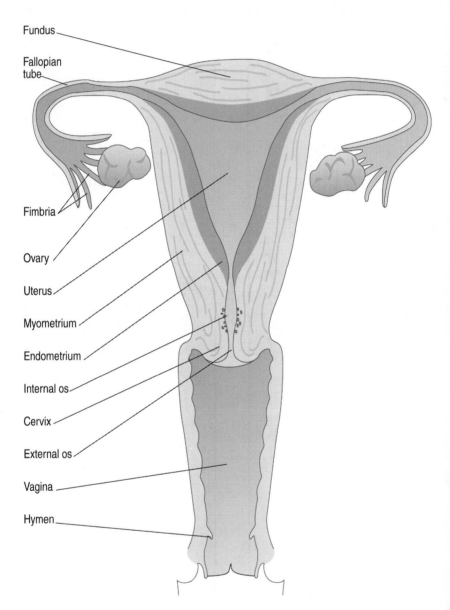

Female reproductive tract

Vaginal discharge

❖ Vaginal discharge occurs, and changes, throughout your menstrual cycle.

❖ Each menstrual cycle starts with a period, which lasts for about 5 days. You will need to use external sanitary pads or internal tampons to protect your clothing.

❖ After that, your vagina will probably appear to be quite dry for a few days, before fertile mucus is produced at the neck of your womb *(cervix)*.

❖ Mucus is cloudy at first then goes clear and stretchy, appearing just like egg white.

❖ After egg release, the mucus gets thicker and your vagina becomes drier, though you'll still have a general moistness to keep you comfortable.

❖ It's perfectly normal to have a clear or slightly white and occasionally watery vaginal discharge, which stains your knickers and doesn't really smell.

❖ But, if the discharge seems unusual, heavier or smells, it's wise to get tested at a GUM/STI clinic in case you've caught a sexually transmitted infection.

Diary keeping

❖ Keeping a diary can be useful.

❖ It can help you to predict accurately when your next period will arrive.

❖ Many times throughout your life you'll be asked for the date of the first day of your most recent period. So it's wise to keep a note in your diary each month to check the length of your menstrual cycle *(cycle).* This helps to assess your fertile times and whether your body is working as it should.

❖ To measure your cycle length in days, you count the number of days from the *first* day of your period, until the day before the *first* day of your *next* period.

❖ Sometimes your period might be longer or shorter than other times, as might the length of your menstrual cycle.

❖ The number of days in a calendar month can vary, so that's why it's a good idea to count the days by looking at calendar dates rather than guess when you think your next period should come.

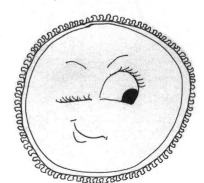
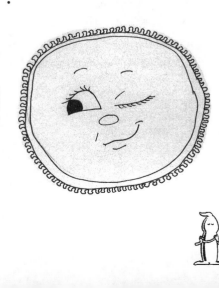

Other changes during puberty

❖ You'll continue to grow in height and weight.

❖ Your figure will start to change with your breasts growing, your hips getting wider, your waist becoming more defined; and you might develop a wiggle as you walk!

❖ Your general body odour may change slightly and you'll gradually become more inquisitive about sex and its mysteries.

❖ You'll probably start to explore your body and start to masturbate.

❖ Masturbation won't make you blind, deaf or drive you mad as people used to say in olden days!

❖ You may become interested in make-up, fashion, music, members of the opposite sex and the appearance of your body.

Sexuality

❖ You may wonder, at some stage, about your sexuality and the people you find attractive.

❖ You might not be attracted to members of the opposite sex but to members of your own or even, to both sexes.

❖ *For further information on sexuality see page 118.*

Menstrual cycle and weight

❖ If you're under or overweight for your age and height your menstrual cycle could be affected.

❖ Your periods may become irregular or perhaps stop until you return to your correct weight.

Cervical maturity

❖ Even if you appear physically mature by your mid teens, your reproductive organs, in particular the neck of your womb *(cervix)* takes until you're about 23 years of age to mature.

❖ Therefore, if you have sex, particularly under this age you'd be wise to use condoms to protect it from infection.

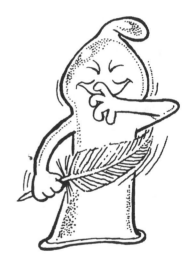

Adolescent development

- You may think that all adults are stupid and don't have a clue how you feel. This is just part of your development.
- You might think you can't talk to any of them. Don't forget they've all gone through similar confusing years, too. They really aren't stupid aliens from outer space!
- They know more about the ways of the adult world. They'd like to help you avoid many of the mistakes they made when they were your age.
- You never know, you might even grow to like them if you give them a chance!
- They'll be happy to help if they know the answers to your questions.
- If you're too shy to talk to your parents or another adult you know well, try asking other people; for example your teacher, School Nurse, youth worker, Doctor, Practice Nurse, trusted aunt, uncle, older brother, sister, cousin or family friend.
- You may prefer to find information by talking to friends, reading books, watching films, or drop into your local Family Planning Clinic where the staff are clued up about sex.
- You'll find that there's a lot more to having sex than just the physical act of intercourse and that there's another side to it.
- You'll learn about the risk of contracting sexually transmitted infections and of unplanned pregnancy in addition to the fun, joy and pleasure of sex.
- By looking after yourself and asking the right questions, sex will also be enjoyable and give you pleasure.
- Remember, though, that with sex you have responsibilities: to your partner as well as yourself.
- It is wrong for an adult to interfere with you sexually. If this has happened or is happening to you, you must tell someone, <u>whatever</u> they say, even if you're scared, so you get help for it to stop.
- *For further information on abuse see page 121-132.*

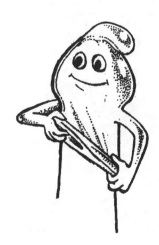

SEXplained...® © 1999 Helen Knox

Smoking

- ❖ There are one or two very good reasons not to smoke!
- ❖ Smoking is, as you'll probably know, bad for your health.
- ❖ Each time you smoke a cigarette hundreds of chemical reactions take place throughout your body.
- ❖ Apart from smelling like an old ashtray with bad breath, there's a strong link between smoking and cancer of the lungs, heart disease, bronchitis, shortness of breath, emphysema, leg ulcers, bladder, stomach, mouth and throat cancer, strokes, high blood pressure and lots more.

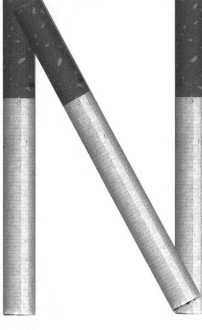

- ❖ **In women**, smoking is linked to cancer of the cervix.
- ❖ **In men**, it's linked to reduced sperm count *(reduced fertility)* and later in life, with impotence *(the persistent inability to get and keep an erection, sufficient for intercourse)*.
- ❖ Would you choose to gamble with your ability to have good sex for many years?
- ❖ Therefore not smoking could improve your sex life!

- ❖ Smoking ages your skin, so by the time you're about 30, you might look about 50 years old!
- ❖ Smoking can also lead to incontinence of urine and of faeces.
- ❖ If you smoke and want help to give up, ask your GP for advice and referral; otherwise, just quit!
- ❖ It may be hard to stop smoking, but living with long term discomfort because of it, is much harder and more painful than the craving for nicotine.
- ❖ Smoking other drugs is illegal and can have damaging effects on your body and your sex life.
- ❖ The choice is yours, you only have one life, so why damage it with a dirty, expensive habit, which may cause years of suffering if you continue? It seems daft!

How can smoking cause high blood pressure?

❖ There are several causes of high blood pressure *(hypertension)*. Commonly it's due to the gradual build up of atheroma *(fatty substances)* on the lining of your arteries and veins. This causes blood to flow less freely along them and your heart has to pump more forcefully to send the same amount of blood around your body.

❖ Think about it another way. When a house is built, the plumber instals clean pipes and water flows freely to your bath, washing machine, sink etc.

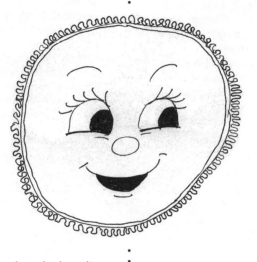

❖ Gradually tough scale deposits inside the pipes, as in your kettle, causing them to fur up and block.

❖ As you get older, depending on what you eat and your general lifestyle, blood or fat cells stick to the lining of your arteries and veins causing rough areas of atheroma to develop which can form a clot and block them.

❖ Due to the extra pressure at which your heart pumps, the clot may be pushed off its resting place and travel around your body.

❖ If it lodges in your brain, it causes a stroke *(CVA or cerebro vascular accident)* in the muscle of your heart it causes a heart attack *(myocardial infarction);* in your lungs it causes a pulmonary embolism; and in your calf muscle, it causes a DVT *(deep vein thrombosis)*.

❖ Smoking is a major factor which increases the stickiness of your blood and greatly increases your risk of developing problems.

Weight and dieting

- ❖ You may become conscious of your weight and your diet. This may be influenced by the fashion industry – from pictures you see of *super-models* in magazines – and want to copy.

- ❖ Some young people develop anorexia *(almost stop eating)* or become bulimic *(make themselves sick after they eat a meal)* to keep their weight low.

- ❖ Many young women have the mistaken belief that men prefer skinny women or that they'll be more popular if they look like some fashion models.

- ❖ What you may not realise is that most men actually *prefer* a woman who has some *padding* on her and aren't particularly attracted to the *walking skeletons* of high fashion.

- ❖ Since this can affect young men too, it's important to realise that a certain amount of fat is *essential* for healthy growth and development.

- ❖ Dieting or weight loss regimens whilst you're young could harm your development if you deprive it of essential food and nutrients when your body's meant to be growing.

- ❖ These are particularly important for healthy bones and regularity of periods.

- ❖ You should only diet if a Doctor says you're overweight and that it's of medical concern.

- ❖ Any dieting should then be under their supervision, to make sure that you don't do more harm to yourself by dieting than by being overweight in the first place.

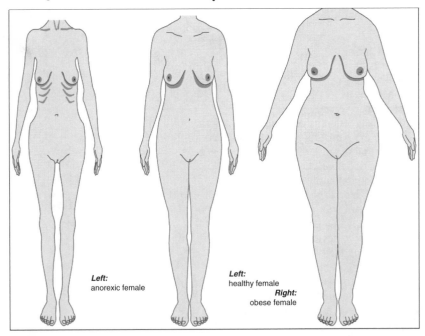

Left:
anorexic female

Left:
healthy female
Right:
obese female

I feel fat and I look gross

I'd look better if I was thinner

I've put on tons of weight

I'll go on a diet

The binge-starve cycle

Binge

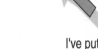

I've lost half a stone.
I look great - even though I'm hungry

I shouldn't have eaten that

I've stopped losing weight and
can't stop thinking about food
- all the time

One piece of cake won't hurt

It's her birthday -
I'm going to have fun.
I may meet someone sexy
at the party.

STARVE   BINGE

The Binge-Starve Cycle

Young Women's Changes & Women's Worries

Breast examination

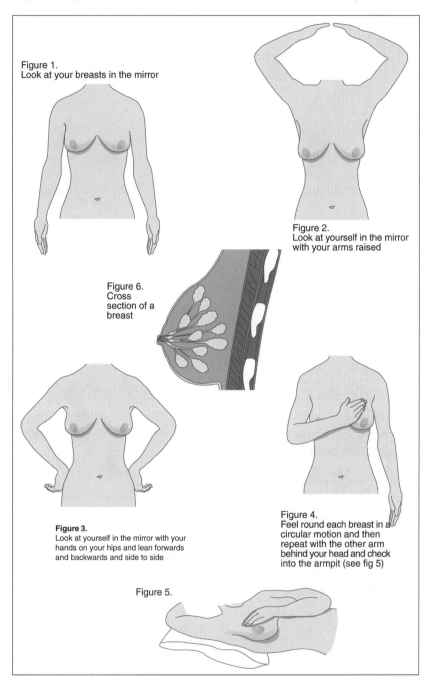

Figure 1.
Look at your breasts in the mirror

Figure 2.
Look at yourself in the mirror with your arms raised

Figure 6.
Cross section of a breast

Figure 3.
Look at yourself in the mirror with your hands on your hips and lean forwards and backwards and side to side

Figure 4.
Feel round each breast in a circular motion and then repeat with the other arm behind your head and check into the armpit (see fig 5)

Figure 5.

SEXplained...® © 1999 Helen Knox

Breast self-examination (BSE)

- ❖ It's sensible for all men and women to be *breast aware*.
- ❖ WOMEN and MEN should check their breasts regularly using the same technique.
- ❖ Partners can check each other's breasts.
- ❖ You may be shown other techniques but they all aim to check your vulnerable areas.
- ❖ You should know the look, shape and texture of your breasts.
- ❖ Breast cancer affects 1 woman in 12 in the UK.
- ❖ It's rare for men, but not unknown.
- ❖ 9 out of 10 lumps found, are not malignant – *ie. they are benign/ non-cancerous* – so, if you find a lump, act quickly and let a Doctor check it out.
- ❖ Either visit your GP or go to a Family Planning/Well Woman Clinic.
- ❖ In the UK, women aged 50 to 65 are automatically invited for free mammography *(special breast X-ray)* every 3 years.

What should I look for when I check my breasts?

Watch for:

- ❖ any changes to the usual look or feel of your breasts.
- ❖ any change to your nipple(s) and any discharge or secretion from them.
- ❖ any change in the direction your nipple(s) point.
- ❖ any puckering or swelling of your breast skin.
- ❖ any bulges in your breast contour.
- ❖ 'orange peel' skin, dimpling or tethering – *ie. as if something is stuck to the inside of it.*
- ❖ any swelling of your upper arm or armpit.

Basic technique

Looking at yourself in the mirror:

❖ stand upright, then lean forwards, then tilt sideways with your arms by your sides.
❖ put your hands on your head – to stretch the breast tissue – and repeat looking, moving and checking as before.
❖ place your hands on your hips and repeat viewing, move and check again, as before.

Figure 1.
Look at your breasts in the mirror

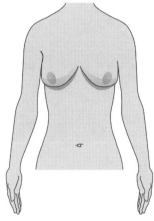

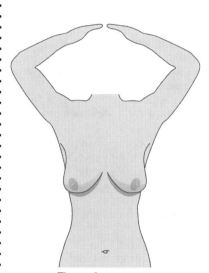

Figure 2.
Look at yourself in the mirror with your arms raised

Then

❖ Be comfortable and relaxed whilst checking.
❖ In a bath or lying on the bed – wherever you're most comfortable. With one arm stretched behind your head, feel your opposite breast in a firm but gentle manner, with the flat of your other hand.

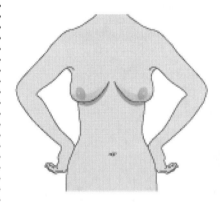

Figure 3.
Look at yourself in the mirror with your hands on your hips and lean forwards and backwards and side to side

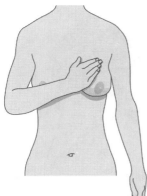

Figure 4.
Feel round each breast in a circular motion and then repeat with the other arm behind your head and check into the armpit (see fig 5)

❖ You will find lumps the first time you check, as your breasts are made up of many glands, surrounded by fat.
❖ These lumps and bumps form a base line from which you can notice any changes.
❖ When you make *breast awareness* part of your routine health care, the stress of regular checking is reduced.
❖ If in doubt, ask your Doctor or Family Planning/Well Woman Clinic to check them for you.

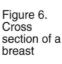
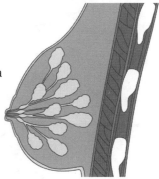

Figure 6.
Cross section of a breast

❖ Start by squeezing your nipple and look for fluid coming out.
❖ Feel in a *Catherine wheel* motion around your nipple area with your hand, round and round the breast area and up into your armpit.
❖ All this time, be aware of the lumps you are feeling.

Figure 5.

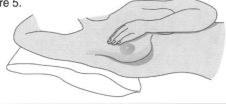

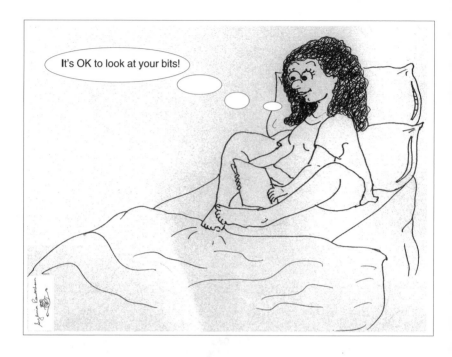

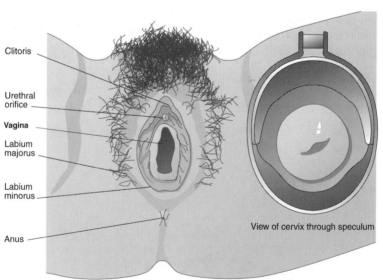

Illustration of female genitalia

What's my clitoris and where is it?

❖ Your clitoris is a small area of erectile tissue situated at the front of your genital area *(vulva)* which is covered by a little hood of skin.

❖ It sits just infront of your urine passage *(urethra)* before the entrance to your vagina.

❖ It has a large supply of blood vessels and nerve endings, which make it very sensitive to touch.

❖ It swells in size and becomes erect when you're sexually aroused, just as a penis gets larger and hard when a man is sexually aroused.

❖ It would have developed into a penis if you'd been a boy instead of a girl.

❖ Like your clitoris, the tip of a penis is sensitive. But the nerve endings of your clitoris are concentrated into a smaller area – hence its *super-sensitivity* when touched.

❖ To help you learn about your anatomy, have a look at yourself in a mirror and explore your genital area *(vulva)*.

I've heard about the *G-spot.* What is it and where can I find mine?

❖ While the term G-spot was popularised by the pop song it doesn't appear in general anatomy text books.

❖ The area is mythical and not so much a physical but psychological area for sexual arousal.

❖ In women it's said to be about 1-1½ inches inside the vagina underneath the bladder; and for men, below the bladder, in the rectum, where the nerve endings change. The muscle in this area is said to be slightly thicker and rubbing it gently is said to be pleasurable.

❖ Not everyone finds it, so don't worry. You can still have perfectly good sexual arousal and orgasm without experiencing the amazing, but possibly mythical, G-spot.

❖ No two orgasms are the same anyway and no two people are the same, so don't start worrying about whether you have a G-spot or not.

❖ Worrying about your anatomy will spoil your enjoyment. Simply enjoy sex safely when you have it.

> *My sentiments exactly.*
> *I feel honoured that they named this spot after me!*
> **Robbie Gee**
> Actor/Comedian

Why do I get wet down below when I think of sex?

❖ Just as young men get erections to show they're sexually aroused *(turned on)*, when you're sexually aroused you make a *welcoming fluid* so that a penis can slip into your vagina easily and painlessly.

❖ Sometimes foreplay *(heavy petting)* is necessary to make this moisture appear.

❖ If you feel hurried or pressured into sex, it's unlikely to flow!

❖ Just because you're wet, it doesn't mean you HAVE to have sex or necessarily WANT to have sex, just that you're becoming aroused!

What is my vagina?

❖ It's a self cleansing passage, between your external genital area and your cervix and womb.

Where is it?

❖ Your vagina is situated in your genital area *(vulva)* between your anus and your urine passage *(urethra)*.

❖ It has a dead end and is only linked to your womb *(uterus)* – not to your bladder or your bowels. So no urine or faeces *(poo)* can leave your body through it.

❖ *See the illustration of female anatomy on page 43.*

What's my hymen?

❖ Your hymen is a very thin layer of skin, which almost covers the entrance to your vagina. As you grow up it may stretch without you realising.

❖ Sometimes it doesn't stretch but is broken or torn when you first insert a tampon or finger. It may stretch during certain athletic movements.

❖ It's broken when you have sex for the first time *(lose your virginity)*.

❖ This may or may not make you bleed a little bit.

If I break it, can it be repaired?

❖ It's possible for a hymen to be repaired surgically, but it's not common practice to do so.

What does the word *virgin* mean?

Virgin means:

❖ being the first or happening for the first time.

❖ a person who has never had sexual intercourse.

If I lose my virginity, how can I find it again?

❖ You can't get your virginity back after you've lost it.

❖ That's why you should be sure you *really* want to lose it before giving it away when you have sex for the first time.

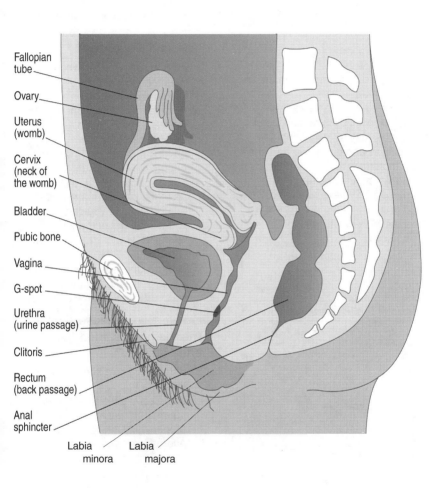

Fallopian tube
Ovary
Uterus (womb)
Cervix (neck of the womb)
Bladder
Pubic bone
Vagina
G-spot
Urethra (urine passage)
Clitoris
Rectum (back passage)
Anal sphincter
Labia minora
Labia majora

Female reproductive organs

Will I lose my virginity if I ride a man's bicycle or a horse?

❖ No, you won't lose your virginity by riding a bicycle.
❖ Although there are male and female saddles, the male saddle doesn't have anything which could penetrate you.
❖ The lady's saddle is wider and is designed to be more comfortable for women.
❖ There's a possibility that with some athletic movements your hymen may stretch, eg. horse riding, gymnastics and perhaps with certain Yoga positions.
❖ However, just because your hymen may have stretched, it doesn't mean you aren't still a virgin – particularly if you haven't had sex.

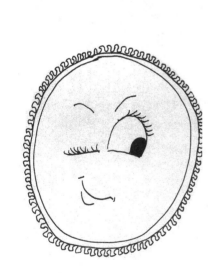

When do girls start their periods?

❖ Girls start their periods between the ages of 9 and 16.

When will I have my first period, become fertile and able to have a baby?

❖ It's impossible to tell when you will start your period.
❖ You could, however, become fertile and get pregnant from just *before* your first period.
❖ Don't think that because you haven't had a period you can't get pregnant. You can!
❖ This is because your egg is released *before* your period, not after. Because you can't tell when your first egg will be released, you can't tell, for sure, when your period will start.
❖ Many young women get caught out by this and become pregnant before they ever have a period.

I'm worried because all my friends have started theirs and I haven't?

❖ Wait until you're about 16 or 17, then see your GP who may do some simple tests to make sure your hormones are working properly.
❖ Alternatively the Family Planning Clinic Doctors and Nurses can advise you.
❖ Many Family Planning Doctors are gynaecologists *(specialists in women's health and medicine)* so they're good to talk to about things like this. They will listen to your fears and give good advice.

Is it common to have irregular periods?

❖ Many young women have irregular periods in the first few years.

❖ Many continue to have irregular periods for many years, although they many settle into a regular pattern.

❖ There is also a common condition called polycystic ovary syndrome *(PCOS)* which causes irregular bleeding cycles and a few other side effects, such as excess hairiness.

❖ Taking the Pill can help control irregular bleeding, as long as the woman is otherwise medically fit.

❖ If you're worried about your periods you should seek medical advice from your GP or Family Planning Clinic.

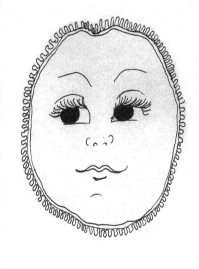

Should I use tampons or sanitary pads/towels when I have my periods?

❖ The decision about which type of protection to use is up to you.

❖ Each has their use. Sometimes you may choose a tampon (internal sanitary protection) and other times you may choose a pad.

❖ Your choice may depend upon what you're wearing, where you're going and how heavy your flow is that day.

❖ If you use tampons, it's important not to leave them in for more than the recommended 8 hours. Don't use a tampon of greater absorbency than you need. Many women change their tampons 3-4 hourly.

❖ Don't use tampons if you have a vaginal infection or an abnormal discharge.

❖ Some women use more absorbent tampons than they need, thinking that they can then leave them in longer, but it's not recommended.

❖ Stale tampons become smelly and there's then the possibility of bacterial *(germ)* growth in the vagina.

❖ Tampons should be removed before you pass urine to ensure that you empty your bladder properly. This will help you to prevent cystitis *(inflammation of the lining of your bladder)*.

❖ Pads should be changed as often as necessary to be comfortable.

Toxic shock syndrome (TSS)

❖ Although this condition is very rare it is something you should be aware of.

❖ TSS is an infection caused by the bacteria staphylococcus aureus.

❖ If tampons are left inside your vagina for a long time *(or forgotten)*, in the presence of the bacteria, they can alter the normal conditions in your vagina and cause problems.

❖ TSS can cause headache, sore throat, aching muscles and joints, high temperature, a rash, dizziness, diarrhoea and even coma from blood poisoning *(septicaemia)* which is a life-threatening condition and has to be treated quickly with antibiotics, probably in hospital.

❖ The use of sanitary towels rather than tampons on light flow days may be helpful and does not carry the same risk.

❖ It is advisable to use tampons with an applicator or wash your hands before and after inserting your tampon.

❖ Many women have changed from using tampons to sanitary pads or towels to avoid the risk of toxic shock syndrome.

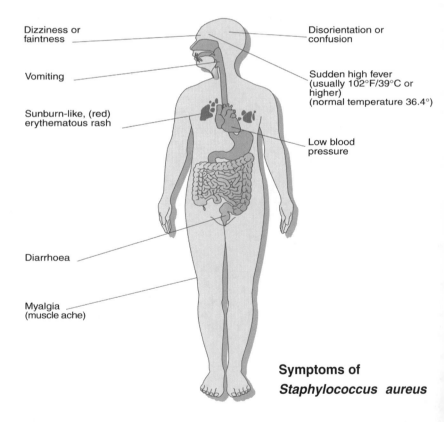

Dizziness or faintness

Vomiting

Sunburn-like, (red) erythematous rash

Diarrhoea

Myalgia (muscle ache)

Disorientation or confusion

Sudden high fever (usually 102°F/39°C or higher) (normal temperature 36.4°)

Low blood pressure

Symptoms of *Staphylococcus aureus*

Will I bleed when I have sex for the first time?

❖ Some people believe that bleeding the first time you have sex proves you're a virgin. That's not true because not all women bleed when they first have sex, and you may be one of them.

If I do bleed, how much will it be?

❖ You should only bleed a little if you bleed at all – when you first have sex.
❖ The bleeding shouldn't continue.

Is it OK to have sex during a period?

❖ Yes, it's OK.
❖ There are no rules about it and it's down to personal preference.
❖ There's nothing dirty or shameful about having your period.
❖ Some women feel more sexy during their period while others don't want anyone to see or know anything about it.
❖ *Generally*, the risk of pregnancy is less at this time, although the risk of infection is higher.
❖ It's equally OK not to want sex during your period.
❖ Your vagina and the neck of your womb *(cervix)* may feel more tender so you may choose to have sex in a position where you're more in control of the depth of penetration.
❖ Some women like to use the contraceptive cap *(diaphragm)* as additional protection to hold back their flow of blood.
❖ Others prefer to place a towel underneath themselves to protect bedding or furniture.

❖ Sex is *never* compulsory. Don't do anything you feel uncomfortable about just to please someone else.
❖ The main rule about sex is that whatever you get up to should be by mutual consent *(agreement)* and not harm anyone else.
❖ In some countries, people still believe that women are unclean during their period and their men won't go near them at this time.
❖ Sometimes it's used as an excuse to have sex elsewhere. This has obvious dangers for sexually transmitting infection if the man returns to their regular partner after having casual sex elsewhere.
❖ As men learn more about women's health and their own risks when they have multiple sexual partners, attitudes change.
❖ Furthermore, since most men wouldn't like their mother or sister to be treated with such disrespect, it would be wise not to cheat on your partner for such a reason.

If my Mum gets ill with her periods, will I too?

❖ No, not necessarily.
❖ Girls often copy *role models* and think they're expected to feel ill too, but this isn't usually the case. There could be many other reasons for feeling ill.

SEXplained...® © 1999 Helen Knox

Heterosexual sex

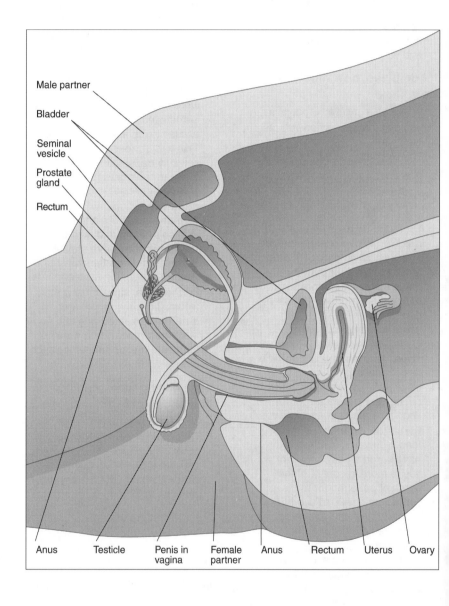

Male partner

Bladder

Seminal vesicle

Prostate gland

Rectum

Anus Testicle Penis in vagina Female partner Anus Rectum Uterus Ovary

What's contraception?

❖ Contraception is a method used by a man or a woman to prevent a pregnancy.

Why is it important for men/women to know about contraception before we first have sex/make love?

❖ It is important to know about contraception if you want to avoid unplanned pregnancy; or you don't want to catch a sexual infection.

❖ Sex is not always as simple as it appears in the movies. So-called roll models don't always provide us with good examples of how to behave.

❖ They don't tell you about pregnancy or catching an infection.

❖ If you consider yourself mature enough to start having a sexual relationship, you should be fully aware that there's much more to healthy sex than just doing it for pleasure. You should take responsibility for your sexual health.

❖ Apart from pregnancy and sexually transmitted infection, there could be serious side effects, physical and emotional, from having sex.

❖ As a young man you should be aware that if you make a girl pregnant – and she continues with the pregnancy – YOU will have to pay money to her for your child every week until s/he leaves full-time education. This could be until they are 25 years of age, so all of this is very important for young men. It's a huge commitment and not one to be taken lightly.

❖ If a young couple doesn't use contraception correctly and consistently, it's extremely common for girls to get pregnant the first time they have sex.

❖ Although a natural occurrence, pregnancy can be dangerous for a woman's health.

❖ Condoms, alone, don't always offer enough protection, particularly when neither of you is practised at putting them on a penis or keeping them on during sex.

❖ Why not share the responsibility and use the *Double Dutch* approach - ie. routinely use condoms AND another method of birth control. So called because it is widely practised in Holland. The Dutch now have the lowest unplanned pregnancy and sexually transmitted infection rates in Europe.

❖ By using the *Double Dutch* approach you can then relax and enjoy each other without the added anxiety of an unplanned pregnancy or risk of infection.

❖ Always seek advice if you're worried that you might be pregnant because you didn't use your method of contraception correctly.

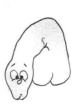
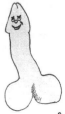

Where can I get contraception?

Contraception is freely available, in the UK, from:

- any Family Planning/Reproductive Health or Brook Advisory Clinic .
- most family Doctors *(GP's)*.
- some GUM clinics *(genito-urinary medicine, also known as STD/ STI or sexually transmitted disease clinics)* at special times.
- many areas have special clinics for young people under the age of 25.
- some private clinics provide it, for a fee.
- *for further information on private clinics see page 182.*

What should we know about contraception?

- In addition to the condom, which should be used routinely for safer sex, there are many methods of contraception. Only celibacy is 100% safe.

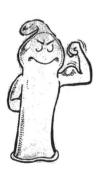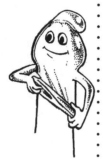

The main methods include:

(a) the combined pill *(the Pill or COC)*.

(b) the progestogen only pill *(mini-pill or POP)*.

(c) the injection *(eg. Depo Provera)*.

(d) the intra-uterine contraceptive device *(IUCD/IUD)* or coil, of which there are many varieties.

(e) the intrauterine system *(IUS)* called Mirena®. Mixture of a coil with the mini-pill built into one. *(Launched in the UK in 1995)*

(f) implants eg. Norplant®, a 5 year contraceptive which is inserted under the skin of the forearm.

(g) female barrier methods such as the Dutch cap *(diaphragm)* which fits along the top of the vagina and covers the neck of the womb *(cervix);* or the cervical cap, which just fits over the cervix.

(h) advice on natural family planning *(safe period)* or referral to a specialist teacher of this method.

(i) referral for male sterilisation *(vasectomy)*.

(j) referral for female sterilisation.

(k) the female condom *(Femidom®/ Reality®)* a barrier method.

(l) the male condom. Used either for contraception or in addition to another contraceptive method ie. for *safer sex.*

(m) Emergency Contraception *(post-coital contraception)* ie. to be taken after sex.

(n) information about the use of Persona®, a mini-computer which can work out your safe times. To use it effectively, you need to understand how to use it – and your body very well. It isn't available free at clinics but can be bought at selected chemists. It is not suitable for all women.

(o) other methods may be used by different countries.

❖ Throughout your life you might try several of these methods, not just one or two.

❖ Each has its advantages and disadvantages. No single method is likely to suit you for life.

❖ To feel happy about using contraception effectively, you should always have a choice.

❖ Different methods of contraception are advised at different times or with certain medical conditions.

❖ *Men should understand how each method works. Taking responsibility for understanding how contraceptive methods work is important for men and women alike as each must/may rely on the other to prevent unwanted pregnancy. Withdrawal or 'pulling out' is not a reliable method of contraception and is not recommended.*

In today's changing times, don't listen to those words...

"I'll be careful, you're safe, I'm clean, you can't get pregnant etc."

Only YOU can truely keep you safe.

So next time the subject of SEX comes up, think about it – make sure YOU are really ready and always, always protect yourself.

Carole Pyke

What else is on offer?

In the UK clinics also offer:

❖ free pregnancy testing.

❖ pre-pregnancy advice.

❖ advice and counselling about rape, impotence, premature ejaculation, and other common sexual worries.

❖ referral for unwanted pregnancy counselling.

❖ post-abortion support and counselling.

❖ breast checks for women of all ages. They will teach you how to be *breast aware*.

❖ routine cervical *(pap)* smear screening tests for women of 20-64 years of age.

❖ hysterectomy advice and support.

❖ menopause advice/support and referral for HRT *(hormone replacement therapy)*.

❖ relationship counselling.

❖ blood tests for rubella *(German measles)*, sickle cell disease and thalassaemia.

❖ blood pressure and weight checks for both men and women.

❖ advice on testicular health and *testicular self-examination* techniques.

❖ Family Planning Clinics are NOT for *women only*. Some areas have started specific clinics for men.

❖ many young men find it difficult to visit a clinic and talk their problems through. But after attending they wish they'd taken the opportunity before.

❖ there are male Doctors at some clinics if you would prefer to talk to a man.

Do I have to be married or planning a family to go to a Family Planning Clinic?

❖ No, you don't – clinics care for young and old, male and female, married or single without age limit.

❖ Staff don't sit in judgement. They are there to help you. So there's no need to feel shy or scared.

Do they need to see any identification of who I am?

❖ No, they don't. They accept what you say.

How old do I have to be to be seen?

❖ They will see you at any age – even if you're under 16.

If I'm under the legal age of consent, won't they think I'm bad for going to a clinic?

❖ No, they won't.

❖ They're not there to judge you.

❖ They respect you for taking responsibility and the maturity which prompted you to seek advice.

Will they contact the Police, social workers, parents, guardians, hostel workers etc.?

❖ No, no-one is contacted without your permission.

❖ Their only concern is for YOU.

Will they lecture me?

❖ No, they won't.

❖ What you do and how you do it is your business.

❖ Any questions you may have about contraception, safer sex, sexual health – even drugs, drug taking or injecting – can be discussed freely with the Nurse or Doctor.

So, if I inject or use drugs, am I still welcome at the clinics?

❖ Yes, you are.

Will they tell my Doctor if I go to a clinic?

❖ No, they won't. The service is strictly confidential and your Doctor is only contacted with your permission – even though some clinics may encourage you to let them write to your GP.

❖ Remember: the choice is yours and yours alone.

How can I be sure?

❖ If you are THAT worried, give only a contact address. But do make sure you can be contacted *somehow*, just in case.

Must I return to the same clinic where I started?

❖ No, you don't have to return to the same clinic.

❖ If you ask, they can write a transfer note for you to take to another clinic or Doctor about any treatment or method you're using.

❖ However, it's sensible to stay with one provider of care, so that you have continuity of medical care.

❖ Once again, the choice is yours.

Won't they laugh at my problems?

❖ No, they won't. They're only interested in helping you.

Are the Doctors male or female at Family Planning Clinics?

❖ The Doctors are usually female in the clinics because they're aware that the majority of women prefer female Doctors.
❖ If you prefer a male Doctor, you can enquire at reception when you first visit.
❖ The Doctors are all specialists in Family Planning with consider-able medical experience in this field.

How much does it cost?

❖ All NHS services and supplies are FREE of charge in the UK.

Can I just go to the clinic for condoms?

❖ Yes and they're free in the UK.
❖ They will usually ask for minimal information in the clinics but some areas offer free condoms at *condom supply points* where no questions are asked.

Where can I find condom supply points?

❖ Each area is different but if you phone your local hospital and ask for the Family Planning Office, they should be able to tell you what your area offers.
❖ BUT, remember, condoms are also available at all Family Planning and GUM/STI Clinics in the UK, FREE of charge.

Why is it called a clinic when I'm not ill?

❖ Good question! Clinic means *centre at which advice and assistance in matters of health, hygiene, maternity etc. are given*.

If I have or have had many partners am I still welcome?

❖ Yes, of course.
❖ They won't judge your lifestyle or lecture you in any way.

What may a clinic need from me?

❖ You'll always be asked to give the date of the FIRST day of your last period.
❖ If that's today then say so, otherwise try and work out the date before you're seen.
❖ If you want a pregnancy test, they need something to test! So, take a sample of that day's urine *(wee)* for testing.
❖ The first *wee* is the most concentrated but other samples can usually give a reliable result.
❖ You don't need a special container. A clean jar or bottle will do and only a few drops are needed.

Can I take a friend or an interpreter with me?

❖ Yes you can. Having company can also help make you less nervous.
❖ Some clinics have interpreters but it helps the clinic staff, too, if English isn't your first language.

Will they show me how to use whatever they give me?

❖ Yes, they teach you how to use your contraceptive method(s) properly and make sure you understand what to do if things go wrong.

❖ If you are ever in any doubt, PLEASE ASK FOR HELP.

❖ Even if your clinic runs by appointment rather than letting you just walk in to be seen without appointment, you don't need an appointment to ask for help.

❖ Alternatively you could phone for advice, when the clinic is open.

Are there any help lines I can ring for advice?

❖ You can ring any Family Planning or Brook Advisory Clinic and ask to speak to a Doctor or Nurse.

❖ Details of clinics can be found in the phone book or at the library.

❖ You can ring and ask to speak to your GP or Practice Nurse.

❖ Your Pharmacist *(chemist)* can also help you.

❖ You can also see any GP in the country who offers contraceptive services – even if they're not your own GP.

❖ *For further information about contraceptive help-lines see* *page 182*

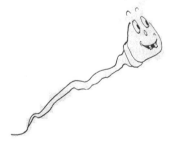

What does having an internal examination involve?

❖ It involves a gentle examination of your genital area by a Doctor.

❖ You may be embarrassed, but the Doctor will only want to make sure that everything is healthy.

❖ They sometimes use a special instrument called a speculum.

❖ This enables the Doctor to look inside your vagina and check that your cervix *(neck of the womb)* is healthy.

❖ Doctors appreciate that some young women find this embarrassing. But it's the only way to check if you really are OK.

❖ There is often a Nurse with you to reassure you and hold your hand. If there's not and you'd like one to be there, just ask.

❖ It's always better to pluck up courage and be sure you're alright, than neglect your health simply because you're embarrassed.

Will it hurt?

❖ No, it won't hurt.

❖ It may be uncomfortable but the more relaxed you are the more comfortable it will be.

❖ Afterwards many people say, *Is that it? I didn't feel a thing. I don't know why I was so scared.*

Do I HAVE to have one?

❖ *An internal examination is **NOT** compulsory at your first visit or before you receive contraception. It may be necessary only if you, yourself, have any health concerns.*

What's a smear (Pap) test?

❖ Regular smear tests are designed to detect any abnormal cell changes at your cervix before they turn into pre-cancerous ones.

❖ It's named after the person who invented it called Papanicolaou.

❖ This is when the neck of your womb *(cervix)* is wiped with a special instrument called a spatula.

❖ The spatula is then wiped across a piece of glass, which is then *fixed* with a special solution and sent to the laboratory.

❖ The laboratory checks the sample to see if any of the cells covering your cervix have changed from the normal pattern.

❖ Sometimes abnormal cells are noticed, which can gradually lead to pre-cancer, if not treated. If that's then left untreated it can lead to *cancer of the cervix,* travel to your womb and on to the rest of your body.

❖ Treatment is now easy, quick and highly successful.

Is cervical cancer a sexually transmitted infection?

❖ Yes cervical cancer is a sexually transmitted infection .... and No.

❖ There are two types of cervical cancer.

❖ One type is considered to be sexually related.

❖ Regular smear tests are made to detect only the sexually related early abnormalities of the cervix, at the entrance to your uterus, which sometimes lead to *squamous cell carcinoma*.

❖ A smear test doesn't, however, check you for sexually transmitted infections, although sometimes one may be detected.

❖ The other, *adenocarcinoma*, is much less common and is more difficult to detect. It usually develops further inside the cervical canal towards the inside of the womb and the cause is less clear.

Smear test

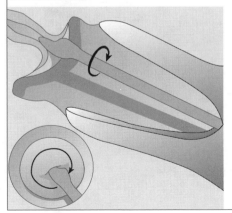

The spatula is inserted into the external os of the cervix and rotated.

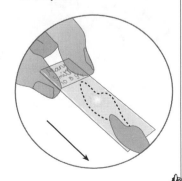

This is then placed flat and drawn along a glass slide to spread the mucus as thinly as possible. This is then fixed and sent to the laboratory for analysis.

When should I have my first smear test?

❖ You should have your first test at 20, unless there are special reasons to have one earlier.

❖ It's important that you're honest with your Doctor or Nurse about when you first had sex, about your sexual history and lifestyle. They are interested only in looking after your future reproductive and sexual health. They're not out to judge you in any way. If you say you were 20 years old but were 10 or 12 when you first had sex, they might guide you about the right time to have your smear test.

Can cervical cancer be prevented?

❖ Yes it can. If abnormalities are found in the early stages, treatment can be given to remove the abnormal cells and prevent this form of cancer developing.

❖ Although having regular cervical smear tests may be embarrassing and you may not like having them, they really are the only way abnormalities can be detected.

❖ You owe it to yourself to have this simple test.

❖ In the UK it is routinely offered to all women between 20 and 65 years of age, FREE.

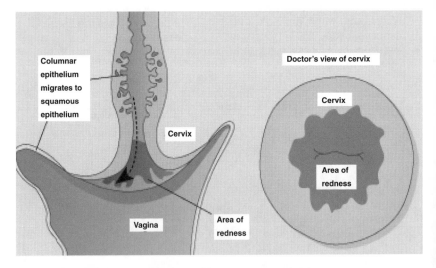

Columnar epithelium migrates to squamous epithelium

Doctor's view of cervix

Cervix

Cervix

Area of redness

Vagina

Area of redness

**Doctors view of a cervix
with inflammation present**

My friend's worried because she had an abnormal smear result and nobody's explained what the different test results mean?

❖ A simple and general translation of smear test results, starting with the most minor follows.

❖ The term CIN stands for *cervical intraepithelial neoplasia* or changes in the cells of the surface of the neck of the womb *(cervix)*.

❖ Cervical cancer develops relatively slowly which is why there is such a high success rate when abnormalities are treated in the first stages of development.

Inadequate – unsatisfactory smear

❖ This may be due to blood or discharge making it difficult to view the other cells easily or the cell sample may have dried too quickly.

❖ These smears should be repeated within 3 months, preferably about two weeks after your period starts.

Negative – normal – no abnormal cells seen on this sample

❖ Repeat after 3 to 5 years if your previous smears have been normal.

❖ Occasionally *thrush, gardnerella, trichomoniasis* or other bugs are detected. However, smear tests do not check for STIs, so you mustn't assume you are clear.

Borderline

❖ Smear should be repeated after 6 months, depending on your medical history.

❖ The majority of these smears return to normal on their own.

❖ If the problem persists, *colposcopy* would be advised.

❖ If you smoke, giving up may help.

❖ HPV *(human papilloma virus)* or genital wart virus, *(the most common STI)* may be associated with these smear results.

Mild dyskaryosis – CIN 1 – low grade changes noted

❖ Repeat smear after 6 months – by then some revert to normal.

❖ CIN1 is often associated with HPV/genital wart virus.

❖ If problem persists, colposcopy is advised.

Moderate dyskaryosis – CIN 2

❖ You would be referred for colposcopy.

Severe dyskaryosis – CIN 3 – high grade changes noted

❖ You would be referred for colposcopy.

What's colposcopy?

❖ Colposcopy is when a specially trained Doctor or Nurse looks at the neck of your womb with a special microscope *(colposcope)* to check for any abnormalities. They paint your cervix with a weak solution of acetic acid *(similar to vinegar)* which *may* sting a little. Abnormal cells show up white and are then viewed more closely.

❖ They may also apply some iodine to your cervix and perhaps take a small sample *(biopsy)* of the abnormal area, to send to the laboratory for further checking. Treatment usually depends on what is seen at colposcopy and/ or as a result of the laboratory test.

Does it hurt?

❖ It's similar to having a smear test but you lie on a special bed and may have the opportunity to see what's happening inside by a special video/TV link.

❖ The biopsy may pinch a little bit but it doesn't last long.

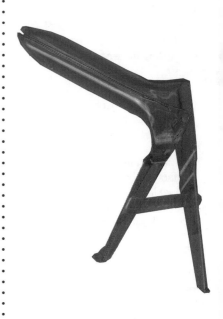

Above:
View of disposable vaginal speculum

Below:
View of spatula and cervical brush

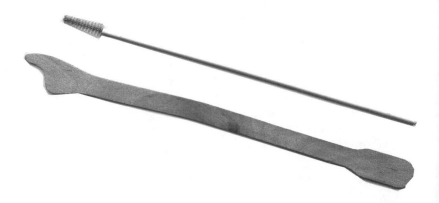

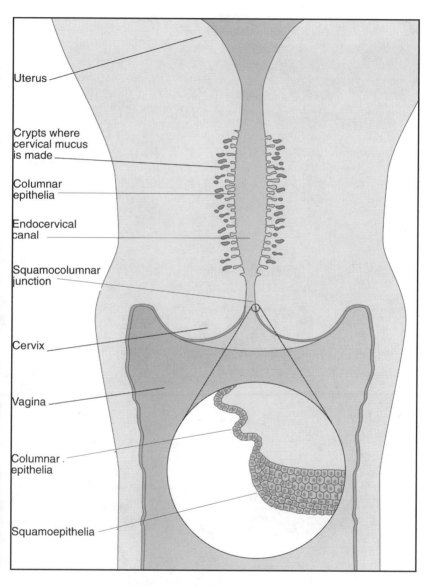

**View of uterine cervix
with enlarged view of squamocolumnar junction**
*This area is also known as the transformation zone and
a smear test aims to check cells sampled from here.
It also shows cervical crytps – where cervical mucus forms.*

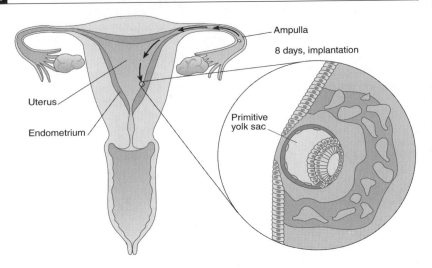

Illustration of fertilisation –
followed by implantation 8 days later

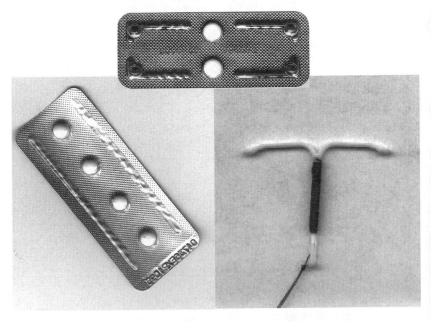

Three types of Emergency Contraception
Schering PC4® – Postinor 2 – IUCD/coil

What's the morning after pill?

❖ The new name for the morning after pill is Emergency Contraception (EC).

Why has it been renamed Emergency Contraception?

❖ That's because it works later than just the morning after unprotected sex.

OK! So what's Emergency Contraception?

❖ Various methods are available.
❖ One method of post-coital contraception *(after sex contraception)*, called Schering PC4®, is four special hormone pills, which you can take within 72 hours of unprotected sex or if you've had an *accident* with your chosen method of contraception, to try and prevent an unplanned pregnancy occurring.
❖ It consists of two hormones – oestrogen and progestogen.

How do I take it?

❖ You take two of these special pills, as soon as possible, followed by another two special pills, exactly 12 hours later.
❖ The first two pills should be taken WITHIN 72 hours *(3 days)* of unprotected sex. The second two should be taken exactly 12 hours later.
❖ Both doses should be taken after you've had something to eat.
❖ Alternatively there's now a progesterone-only method of post-coital contraception which *(unlicensed in the UK at present)* involves taking 20 or 25 special pills followed by 20 or 25 more within 12 hours, started within **72 hours** of unprotected sex. Even though they're a lot of pills to swallow they only contain one hormone and it's a very safe and useful alternative.

❖ In future it's expected to come as single dose pills called Postinor 2. You'd take one Postinor pill, as soon as possible, followed by another Postinor pill, exactly 12 hours later.

What does Emergency Contraception do to my body?

❖ Each of these methods alters the conditions inside your womb to prevent an unplanned pregnancy.

What should I do after I take it?

❖ After taking either of these hormonal methods you should return to using birth control immediately. However, if you take pills, the manufacturer of Schering PC4® recommends that you have no sex or use a barrier method *(condom or cap)* until your next menstrual period. Your doctor may advise you differently.

What if I miss the 72 hours?

❖ If you miss the 72 hours a specially trained Family Planning Doctor may fit an *emergency IUCD/coil*, generally up to 5 days after unprotected sex although in certain circumstances it may be later into your cycle.

Where can I get Emergency Contraception?

❖ The pills are not yet given out in advance or over the counter at a pharmacy, but can be obtained free from all Family Planning Clinics, most GP's, some hospital casualty departments and GUM/STI clinics.

❖ At the GP's you may have to explain to the receptionist why you need an emergency appointment, otherwise you may not be seen until it's too late to prescribe the pills.

❖ Some private clinics offer Emergency Contraception, but you will have to pay for it.

When should I get my period after taking Emergency Contraception?

❖ You should bleed within 3 weeks of taking emergency contraceptive pills.

❖ If you have a lighter bleed than usual or no bleed, see your Doctor to check that you're OK.

Will it make me sick?

❖ You're unlikely to be sick if you take the pills with food. But, the manufacturer of Schering PC4® recommends that if you vomit within 2 hours of taking the first two emergency contraceptive pills you should take the second two and seek medical attention, the same or next day, to obtain more pills or have an emergency IUCD/coil fitted.

❖ Sometimes an anti-sickness tablet is given with the pills (anti-emetic).

How reliable is it?

❖ It's very effective, especially when taken nearer the time you have unprotected sex.

❖ As with any method of contra-ception, you should appreciate that it can fail and should never be used as an alternative to reliable contraception.

❖ It prevents at least 3 out of 4 pregnancies.

Is it suitable for everyone?

❖ If you're pregnant you shouldn't take it.

❖ If you have a migraine at the time you need to take it, you may be prescribed the progesterone only method instead of Schering PC4® – or offered an IUCD.

❖ If you had unprotected sex more than 72 hours ago you may have an emergency coil/IUCD.

How many times can I use it?

❖ There is no limit to the number of times you can have it, although, if you need to use it often, your Doctor may suggest you use a more reliable method of regular contraception, such as the combined Pill or the injection.

❖ If you take it often you may suffer from irregular bleeding.

Will it make my periods heavier or lighter?

❖ Your next period is unlikely to be any different.

❖ However, if it's lighter than usual or you develop tummy pains, tell your Doctor.

❖ There's a small risk it may not work for you in which case, you may become pregnant or develop an ectopic (tubal) pregnancy.

Emergency Contraception

What should I be aware of if my girlfriend's using it?

❖ If you had unprotected sex and didn't bother to use a condom, you should be more responsible and better prepared next time you have sex.

❖ If your condom broke or came off, practise the correct way to wear them and avoid this happening again.

❖ Don't rely on Emergency Contraception instead of a regular method of birth control since it *can* fail.

❖ Go *Double Dutch* and use a reliable method of contraception routinely to protect against pregnancy, AND a condom to protect against infection. This gives much better protection.

❖ If either of you develops an unusual discharge, sores or pains after needing Emergency Contraception, seek a full check-up at a GUM clinic just incase you've caught a sexually transmitted infection.

❖ This is especially important if you were having casual sex or if either of you was unfaithful, while in a regular relationship.

If Emergency Contraception fails to work will it harm the baby?

❖ As far as is known, it won't harm the baby.

❖ But no-one can guarantee a normal baby.

Will Emergency Contraception make me put on weight?

❖ No.

Will it protect me from infection AND pregnancy?

❖ No, just pregnancy.

Will it cause me to have an abortion?

❖ This has been argued extensively around the world and no, it does not cause an abortion.

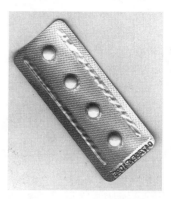

❖ It alters ovulation and changes the conditions in your womb *before* a fertilised egg is able to implant.

Do recreational drugs affect the reliability of Emergency Contraception?

❖ No, they don't.

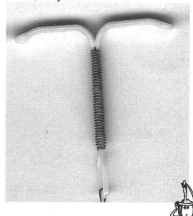

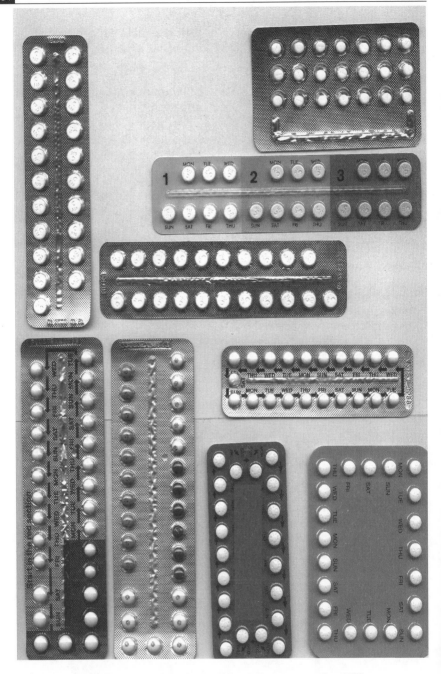

Selection of Combined Oral Contraceptive Pills

What is it?

❖ It's a drug combination of two of the female hormones you already make, oestrogen and progesterone, in the form of progestogen.

How does it work?

❖ It's an oral contraceptive Pill, which fools your body into thinking that you're already pregnant, because pregnant women don't ovulate or release more eggs.

❖ It makes the mucus at your cervix thicker so sperm can't get into your womb; it also changes the conditions in the lining of your womb *(endometrium);* and your fallopian tubes.

❖ This ensures that a steady level of the hormones filter into your bloodstream, to keep your ovaries *(where your eggs are made)* asleep – thereby ensuring that you cannot get pregnant.

How do I take it?

❖ Your active Pill should be taken at the same time every day for, usually 21 days *(some brands have 22 active pills in a packet),* then you take a break for 7, starting your pills again on the 8th day.

❖ Some Pill packets also contain 7 dummy pills, which provide a useful reminder to help you take your pill on the days where you take a break between your active pills. They are known as ED *(every day)* combined oral contraceptive pills.

❖ These ED Pills are taken EVERY day of the year. *(They differ from the mini-pill/POP, which only contains one drug but is also taken every day).*

What if I miss a pill?

❖ Many people think that it takes several months to start releasing eggs again after coming off *The Pill.* This isn't true.

❖ If you miss a pill but take it within **12 hours** from the time it should be taken, you will still be protected.

❖ If, however, it's **over 12 hours** from the time you should have taken your pill, **you will no longer be protected.**

❖ Don't stop the pills.

❖ Continue to take your pills as usual, but use extra protection ie. a condom, cap or not have sex *(abstain)* for the next 7 days.

❖ If those 7 days go into what would have been the 7-day break between packets – don't take the break but start a new packet and take it to the end of the course *(one day at a time).*

❖ At the end of *that* packet, have the 7-day break as usual.

❖ This will not harm you.

❖ During the seven-day break your ovaries start to wake up. If they're not sent back to sleep in time then, there's a risk of an egg being released.

Combined Oral Contraceptive Pill (COC)

Do diarrhoea, vomiting, antibiotics or other prescription drugs affect the Pill?

❖ If you have bad diarrhoea or vomiting, are taking antibiotics or some other prescription medicines *(particularly TB drugs)*, you should assume that protection has been lost.

❖ Extra protection *(or no sex)* is essential during any illness or when taking medication **and** for 7 days afterwards.

❖ If any of that time goes into what would have been your 7 day break between packets, you should start taking the pills, in turn, from the next packet after completing the present packet – and **then** have the normal break *(as before)*.

❖ If you're in any doubt as to which medicines cause problems, check with the doctor who prescribed them, ring any Family Planning Clinic; or ask a Pharmacist.

❖ If you miss two or more pills, seek immediate medical advice because you may require Emergency Contraception.

How reliable is it?

❖ It is extremely reliable if you remember to take it as directed – ie. it can be up to 99.8% effective when taken properly.

❖ Only 2 women in 1,000 are unlucky enough to get pregnant each year, even if they take the Pill properly.

Who can take it?

❖ Generally, it's suitable for fit, healthy young women – particularly non-smokers *(or those who only smoke a little)* aren't very overweight and don't have any serious medical conditions.

Who can't use it?

❖ It's not recommended for young women who:

(a) are pregnant.

(b) have epilepsy – because of interacting drugs. But check with your Doctor.

(c) have high blood pressure *(hypertension)*.

(d) are already pregnant.

(e) get certain types of migraine.

(f) have or have had circulatory problems *e.g. blood clots in your system (thrombosis)*.

(g) are breast feeding.

(h) a) are under 35 and smoke over 40 a day.
b) over 35 years of age and smoke.

(i) have active liver disease *(hepatitis)*.

(j) have cancer of the breast.

(k) have diabetes – if there are other complications.

(l) have unexplained vaginal bleeding.

(m) have sickle cell disease *(a blood disorder)*, but not sickle cell trait.

(n) have tuberculosis *(TB)* – because of interacting drugs.

(o) have severe varicose veins.

(p) are bedridden.

(q) have some other rare medical conditions.

Do I have to have sex to use it?

❖ No, you don't. Few people realise that there are many benefits from taking the Pill apart from preventing pregnancy.

What are the benefits apart from avoiding pregnancy?

❖ If you take it properly. Some of the benefits may include:

(a) fewer acne-type spots *(with some pills)*.

(b) less non-cancerous breast disease.

(c) regular withdrawal bleeds *(periods)*.

(d) less painful periods.

(e) *(generally)* lighter periods.

(f) less anaemia.

(g) no ovulation pain.

(h) less unwanted hair growth.

(i) some protection against cancer of the ovaries and endometrium *(lining of the womb)*.

(j) less endometriosis *(a condition where tissue, similar to the lining of your womb, bleeds (outside your womb) into your pelvic cavity and causes pain)*.

(k) fewer ovarian cysts *(enlarged pus filled sacs on your ovaries similar to acne spots on your face)*.

(l) less troublesome fibroids *(non-cancerous/benign tumours or growths in your uterus)*.

(m) less rheumatoid arthritis.

(n) no anxiety over unwanted pregnancy and it doesn't interfere with sex.

How many years can I take it for?

❖ If you remain fit and well – and don't smoke – you can use it for over 20 years without a break.

❖ If you're a smoker, you'll be taken off it, automatically, by the time you're 35.

Why are smokers taken off the Pill and non-smokers allowed to stay on it?

❖ Smokers are taken off the Pill to protect their health.

❖ Smoking makes your blood more sticky and so can the oestrogen in the combined Pill.

❖ As you get older your risk of having a heart attack or stroke from a sticky blood clot lodging in your heart muscle or your brain increases. This is why you will be advised to stop taking the combined Pill.

❖ If you stop smoking you may be allowed to stay on the combined Pill over the age of 35.

❖ If you're a non-smoker you may be able to stay on it right up until your menopause and then, if you would like, transfer to HRT *(hormone replacement therapy)*.

Should I stop taking the Pill and give my body a break?

❖ No. Your body gets a break from it every four weeks anyway.

❖ By the end of your 7-day break between packets, the drugs are virtually out of your system.

❖ That's why you must use extra protection if you start your next packet late or if you forget to use condoms again.

Will the Pill control my periods?

❖ Yes, it will. Your periods will be regular and you may be able to predict them, right down to the hour they start.

Will it make my periods heavier or lighter?

❖ Generally, the Pill makes your periods lighter and less painful with fewer pre-menstrual symptoms.

Something's going wrong somewhere. I asked this girl if she had protection and she pulled out a knife on me instead of a condom!

Glazz Campbell
Comedian

What should I be aware of if my girlfriend's using it?

❖ You have an interest and a responsibility in understanding about the Pill and how it works to prevent your girlfriend becoming pregnant.

❖ Her outward appearance will not change when she's taking the Pill, so you'll have to trust her to take it properly.

❖ If your girlfriend were to become pregnant, with or without a termination you'd have to deal with the difficult emotions. Without a termination you'd be responsible for paying maintenance for up to 25 years.

❖ There will also be times when you will need to use condoms for protection against pregnancy and routine protection against infection.

❖ The only way to protect yourself in case she hasn't taken it properly is to use a condom routinely for safer sex.

❖ Since most women would find it hard to trust a man saying he was taking the Pill, you should read about how it works, since you also rely on it for protection against pregnancy.

Do recreational drugs affect the Pill's reliability?

❖ No. Not as far as is known.

❖ Drugs can, however, be bad for your long-term physical and mental health and can increase your risk of contracting sexually transmitted infections.

❖ If you dehydrate you are more likely to get thrombosis *(blood clots)*.

Will the Pill make me put on weight?

- You may, temporarily, put on a little bit of weight *(3-4 lbs.)* in the first couple of months due to water retention.
- A little extra weight is safer than pregnancy so, if you do put on weight, don't stop taking your pills. Ask your Doctor about changing to a different variety.
- Try to give it three months before making up your mind that it doesn't suit you. It takes a little time for your body to fully adjust.
- Some women become aware of a slightly nauseous sensation in their throat – but this should wear off soon and you're most unlikely to vomit.
- Again, don't stop taking your pills. Try taking your pill at night instead, so you can sleep through or; take them after breakfast, which may be an easier time to take them routinely.

When does the Pill start to work when I begin to take it?

- You're contraceptively protected from the moment you take your 1st pill on the 1st day of your period.
- If you start it later than day 2 of your period, you need to use extra protection or have no sex *(abstain)* for 7 days. You're safe from pregnancy if you continue to take it properly, thereafter.

Will it protect me from pregnancy AND infection?

- No, it won't. You will still need to use condoms for protection against sexually transmitted infection.
- The barrier of mucus, which forms at your cervix, may slow down the progress of an infection into your womb and tubes, but it won't prevent you from catching it.

Are the effects of the Pill reversible?

- Yes, they are. It's virtually out of your system by the end of your 7-day break.
- But remember: you can get pregnant after that if you have unprotected sex. So use condoms from the day after your last pill, if you don't want to get pregnant.

Is it safe to have sex during my 7-day break?

- Yes you are. As long as you start your next packet of pills on time; you don't have diarrhoea or vomiting; you aren't taking medication which can interfere with the Pill; you're contraceptively protected.
- If in doubt; ask your Family Planning Clinic, ring the Contraceptive Education Service (CES) helpline; or ask your Pharmacist for advice.
- *For further information on the CES see page 182.*

Combined Oral Contraceptive Pill (COC)

If I'm going on holiday and don't want to bleed while I'm away, is there anything I can do?

❖ Yes there is. To avoid your withdrawal bleed (period) – instead of taking your 7 day break between packets of pills/ active pills – simply start your next packet of pills when you finish your present pack – take all of those in turn and *then* take your usual break.

❖ It's OK to do this occasionally, but NOT every month.

When should I call my Doctor?

❖ Despite many precautions to ensure that only women who are medically fit to take it are given the Pill, sometimes complications do occur.

❖ If you notice sudden severe shortness of breath with chest pain, or a painful hot tender swelling in your calf *(lower leg)*, contact your Doctor immediately or Casualty Department in case a blood clot *(thrombosis)* has formed, for which you may need urgent medical treatment.

❖ Thrombosis is very rare but is an important reason why you should be open and honest with whoever takes your and your family's medical history.

❖ When you collect more pills, tell the Doctor about any worries or concerns you may have however minor or silly you think they are.

How old do I have to be to start taking the Pill?

❖ You can start taking the Pill once you have regular, established periods.

Also:

❖ never take unnecessary risks.

❖ check with your Family Planning Clinic or your GP if in doubt about anything.

❖ use extra protection unless you're reliably informed that it's not necessary.

❖ always take the Pill you've forgotten, even if this means taking two pills on one day.

❖ there are many different types of pill. If you think one doesn't suit you, you can always try others until you find the one which is right for you.

Will they show me what to do if I go to a Family Planning Clinic, my doctor, Practice Nurse or Pharmacist?

❖ Whoever gives you the Pill should teach you how it should be taken before you leave the Family Planning Clinic, surgery or chemist.

❖ They should also give you an instruction leaflet to keep as a reference – ie. in case you need to check what you were told at any time.

❖ If, for some reason you're not shown how to take your Pill, ask them to make time to teach you before you leave, so you are sure of what to do.

What to do if you forget your Pill

(This applies to 21 day pill packets
NOT to ED preparations
OR to forgotten mini-pill/POPs)

Missed/forgotten Pill

If you are **late by UP TO 12 hours** from your usual Pill taking time.

Take your missed pill now and your next one on time – continue usual routine.

If you are **late by MORE THAN 12 hours** from your usual Pill taking time.

Take missed Pill now and next one on time – continue usual routine.

BUT – use extra protection (condom or no sex!) for 7 days.

Count the number of remaining Pills in your packet

If 7 or more Pills are left:

have your usual break at the end of your packet.

If less than 7 Pills are left:

do not take your 7 day break between packets but continue into your next packet, without taking a break. Then continue as usual.

if you miss **more than 2 pills in the first 7 days** of the packet and you have unprotected sex, seek medical advice about **Emergency Contraception**.

If more Pills are missed, if you are taking a different type of Pill or **you have any doubts or worries** – call the **Contraceptive Education Service helpline** at the FPA. *(See page 182 for details.)*

SEXplained...® © 1999 Helen Knox

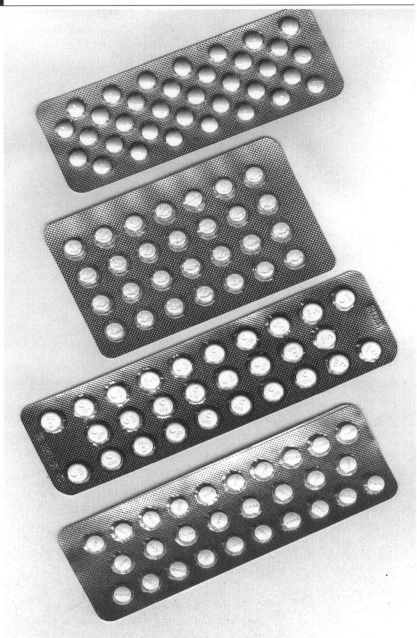

Different types of Progestogen-Only Contraceptive Pills

What is the POP?

❖ The POP or mini-pill as it's known in Family Planning, is an oral contraceptive pill which contains just one hormone – progestogen.

How does it work?

❖ It works by forming a barrier of mucus at your cervix *(neck of your womb)*, so that sperm can't swim through to meet an egg.
❖ It also effects the lining of your womb – and helps to prevent pregnancy.

When or how do I use it?

❖ The pills must be taken EVERY DAY of the year at exactly the same time – without a break.

Will it control my periods?

❖ No, it won't control them at all.
❖ No-one can tell how it will affect your periods.

Will it make my periods heavier or lighter?

❖ Generally, you'll have lighter periods. They may stop.
❖ Some women get irregular light bleeding *(spotting)* in the first few months.
❖ Other women continue to bleed as they did before taking it.

If I forget a mini-pill/POP, what should I do?

❖ If you remember *within three hours* from the time you've decided to take it regularly, just take it and continue as usual.
❖ If you've *forgotten for more than three hours,* continue taking the pill as usual when you remember, but to be safe you must use **extra protection** or have **no sex** *(abstain)* **for 7 days** afterwards.

What if I forget more than one mini-pill/POP?

❖ If you forget two or more pills and have sex, seek immediate medical advice for Emergency Contraception.
❖ If in doubt, ask your Pharmacist.

Do diarrhoea or vomiting affect it?

❖ Yes they do – your protection will be reduced if you have bad diarrhoea or vomiting, especially within 3 hours of taking your pills.
❖ EXTRA PROTECTION is important during illness and with some types of medication.
❖ To be absolutely sure, you should use extra protection for 7 days after you've recovered.

Progestogen-Only Contraceptive Pill (POP)

Do antibiotics or other prescription drugs affect the mini-pill/POP?

- ❖ Drugs for TB and some other drugs can affect it.
- ❖ Antibiotics don't affect it. But if you're worried about other drugs it's always safer to use extra protection before checking with your Family Planning Clinic, Doctor or Pharmacist.

How reliable is the mini-pill/POP?

- ❖ When taken properly it's nearly as reliable as the combined Pill, especially in women over 35.

Will my weight make a difference?

- ❖ If you weigh over 70 kgs you may be advised to take two of these pills, at the same time each day, instead of one a day.

Who's suitable to take it?

- ❖ It's suitable for most women but also if you:
1. are a smoker over 35 years of age.
2. are breast feeding.
3. have high blood pressure.
4. get migraines.
5. are diabetic.
6. have sickle cell disease (*type of blood disease*).
7. if you don't want to take or don't like the combined Pill for any reason.

Who's it NOT suitable for?

- ❖ Most young women are safe to use it but it's not suitable for pregnant women or women with some potentially serious medical conditions.
- ❖ You should discuss with your Doctor if someone in your family has; or if you've had or have:
1. breast cancer.
2. ectopic pregnancy.
3. unusual vaginal bleeding.
4. active liver disease *(hepatitis)*.
5. circulatory or cardiac *(heart)* problems.

For how many years can I use the mini–pill/POP?

- ❖ You can use this excellent method daily, for many years, without worry.

Should I stop using the mini-pill/POP and give my body a break?

- ❖ No, you shouldn't. It's a very safe form of contraception.
- ❖ If you're one of those who stop having periods whilst using it, your Doctor may ask to test your blood after three years and may give you additional hormone treatment for a short while to balance your hormones.

Can I use it safely if I smoke?

- ❖ Yes, you can.
- ❖ If you're taking the combined Pill and smoke, when you reach 35 years of age you'll be transferred automatically to the POP if you still want to use hormonal contraceptive pills.

Do I have to have sex to use it?

❖ No, you don't.

What should I be aware of if my girlfriend's using the mini-pill/POP?

❖ You have an interest and a responsibility in understanding about the POP and how it works to prevent your girlfriend becoming pregnant.

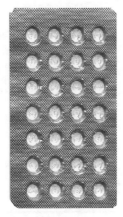

❖ Her outward appearance will not change when she's taking the POP, so you'll have to trust her to take it properly.

❖ If your girlfriend were to become pregnant, with or without a termination you'd have to deal with the difficult emotions. Without a termination you'd be responsible for paying maintenance for up to 25 years.

❖ There will also be times when you will need to use condoms for protection against pregnancy and routine protection against infection.

❖ The only way to protect yourself in case she hasn't taken it properly is to use a condom routinely for safer sex.

❖ Since most women would find it hard to trust a man saying he was taking the mini-pill/POP, you should read about how it works, since you also rely on it for protection against pregnancy.

Do recreational drugs affect the mini-pill/POP's reliability?

❖ No. Not as far as is known.

❖ Drugs can, however, be bad for your long-term physical and mental health and can increase your risk of contracting sexually transmitted infections.

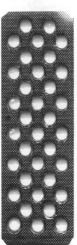

❖ If you dehydrate you are more likely to get thrombosis *(blood clots)*.

Will it make me put on weight?

❖ No, it shouldn't. But if you do put on weight, you could try a different variety of POP, which might suit you better.

Will it protect me from pregnancy AND infection?

❖ No, it won't. You will still need to use condoms for protection against sexually transmitted infection.

❖ The barrier of mucus, which forms at your cervix, may slow down the progress of an infection into your womb and tubes, but it won't prevent you from catching it.

SEXplained...® © 1999 Helen Knox

Are the effects of the mini-pill/POP reversible?

* Yes, they are. It's out of your system after 27 hours.
* But remember: you can get pregnant after that if you have unprotected sex. So use condoms from the day after your last pill, if you don't want to get pregnant.

When does the mini-pill/POP start to work when I begin to take it?

* You're contraceptively protected from the moment you take your 1st pill on the 1st day of your period.
* If you start it later than the second day of your period, you need to use extra protection or have no sex *(abstain)* for 7 days. You're safe from pregnancy if you continue to take it properly, thereafter.

Also:

* never take unnecessary risks.
* check with your Family Planning Clinic or your GP if in doubt about anything.
* use extra protection unless you're reliably informed that it's not necessary.
* always take the pill you've forgotten, even if this means taking two pills on one day and use extra protection *(a condom)* or don't have sex *(abstain)* for 7 days.
* there are many different types of pill. If you think one doesn't suit you, you can always try others until you find the one which is right for you.

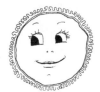

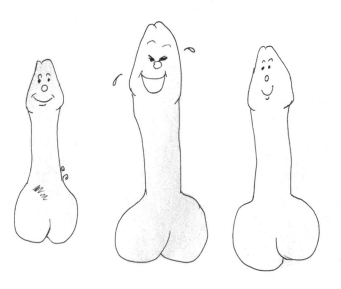

What is injectable contraception?

* It's an extremely effective form of contraceptive.
* It's given by intramuscular injection either monthly *(not yet available in the UK)*, eight weekly or every 12 weeks.
* Some types of injection contain oestrogen and progestogen; some just progestogen.
* Depo-Provera is the most common contraceptive injection used in the UK. It only contains only one drug – progestogen.

How does it work?

* Its action is similar to that of the combined Pill.

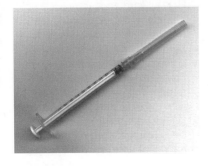

How reliable is this form of contraception?

* It's extremely reliable. It can't fall out, be forgotten *(on a daily basis)* and, it can't split or come off.

Who's suitable to use it?

* It's suitable for most women.

Who's NOT suitable to use it?

* It's not suitable for pregnant women or women with some potentially serious medical conditions.
* You should discuss with your Doctor if you or someone in your family have or has had:
  1. breast cancer.
  2. unusual vaginal bleeding.
  3. active liver disease *(hepatitis)*.
  4. circulatory or cardiac (heart) problems or abnormal blood test results when checking for cholesterol or lipids *(fats)* in your circulation.
  5. depression.

Are there any other benefits from using the injection?

* Yes there are several benefits:
  1. it gives some protection against cancer of the lining of your womb.
  2. it reduces your risk of ectopic *(tubal)* pregnancy.
  3. it reduces your risk of developing ovarian cysts.
  4. it reduces the possibility of having PID *(pelvic inflammatory disease)*.
  5. women with sickle cell disease experience fewer problems than with other methods of contraception.

Injectable Contraception

When or how do I use it?

❖ Depo-Provera is given in the first 5 days of a menstrual cycle and then repeated after 10-12 weeks, for as long as you need contraceptive protection.

When does it start to work?

❖ The injection starts to work as soon as you have it, provided that it's given in the first 2 days of your period.

❖ If you start it between the 3rd and 5th day, you need to use extra protection or not have sex *(abstain)* for 7 days to prevent pregnancy.

Will it control my periods?

❖ No, it won't control your periods.

❖ Over half the women who use it stop having periods or have a very light bleed every few months.

❖ Other women get irregular bleeding. If that happens to you, tell your Doctor so that you can be given additional treatment or shorten the length of time between injections.

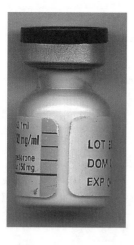

Will it make my periods heavier or lighter?

❖ Periods are generally much shorter and much lighter when using Depo-Provera.

Should I stop using it and give my body have a break?

❖ Not usually.

❖ If you're one of those who stop having periods whilst using it, your Doctor may ask to test your blood after three years and may give you additional hormone treatment for a short while to balance your hormones.

❖ Long term use of this method is widely practised world-wide.

For how many years can I use injectable contraception?

❖ You can take it for many years without worry.

Is it affected by diarrhoea, vomiting or antibiotics?

❖ No, it's not.

What should I be aware of if my girlfriend's using it?

❖ You have an interest and a responsibility in understanding about the injection and how it works to prevent your girlfriend becoming pregnant.

❖ Her outward appearance will not change when she's taking the injection, so you'll have to trust her to take it properly.

❖ If your girlfriend were to become pregnant, with or without a termination you'd have to deal with the difficult emotions. Without a termination you'd be responsible for paying maintenance for up to 25 years.

❖ There will also be times when you will need to use condoms for protection against pregnancy and routine protection against infection.

❖ The only way to protect yourself in case she hasn't taken it properly is to use a condom routinely for safer sex.

❖ Since most women would find it hard to trust a man saying he was taking the injection, you should read about how it works, since you also rely on it for protection against pregnancy.

Do recreational drugs affect the its reliability?

❖ No. Not as far as is known.

❖ Drugs can, however, be bad for your long-term physical and mental health and can increase your risk of contracting sexually transmitted infections.

❖ If you dehydrate you are more likely to get thrombosis *(blood clots)*.

Will it make me put on weight?

❖ No, it shouldn't.

❖ Some women put on weight although some lose weight or stay the same.

❖ No-one can tell how you will react before you use it.

Will it protect me from pregnancy AND infection?

❖ No, it won't. You will still need to use condoms for protection against sexually transmitted infection.

❖ The barrier of mucus, which forms at your cervix, may slow down the progress of an infection into your womb and tubes, but it won't prevent you from catching it.

Is it reversible?

❖ Yes and it's the first method of choice for many young women.

❖ It's out of your system by the 13th week after injection, which is why extra protection is vital if you forget to turn up on time for your injection.

❖ Some women only take a few months to become pregnant after they stop the injection; others take longer. This is because in nature some women are more fertile than others.

❖ Some women experience a delay in re-turn to fertility – but never assume that you will be one of them.

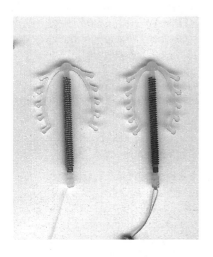

Multiload short   *Multiload*

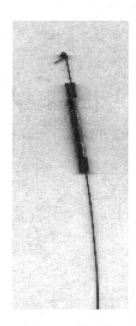

Gyne-Fix

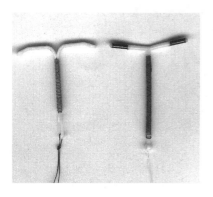

Nova-T   *CuT 380*

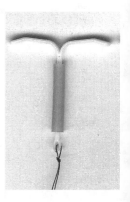

Mirena® - the IUS

Selection of Intra-Uterine Contraceptive Devices and *Mirena®*, the Intra-Uterine System (IUS)

What is the IUCD or coil?

- IUCD means Intra-Uterine Contraceptive Device.
- Some people refer to it as the IUD instead.
- It is a small device, which is inserted into the womb to prevent pregnancy.
- Several different types are available. They're usually made of plastic, contain a small amount of copper and have a small thread, which you can feel at your cervix. *(This helps you to check that it's in place correctly).*

How does it work?

- The copper reduces the number of sperm reaching your fallopian tubes.
- It alters the conditions inside your womb and reduces the chance of fertilisation or of a fertilised egg implanting in your womb.

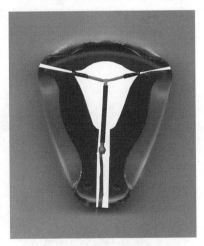

IUCD in position in model uterus

When do I use it?

- It must be inserted by a specially trained Family Planning Doctor or Specialist Nurse under sterile conditions.
- Usually, it's inserted during the first 10 days of a menstrual cycle – although it can be inserted later, as a form of *Emergency Contraception*.

How do I check that it is still there?

- After insertion, you or your partner should check that it's still in place after each period.
- You do this by inserting a clean finger into your vagina and feeling for the thread at your cervix.
- Your cervix is about a full finger's depth into your vagina – it is around hard muscle which feels like the end of your nose – ie. it has a dimple in the centre.
- If you don't feel the thread, assume it has fallen out. You must then use another method of contraception until you can get it checked by your Doctor or Nurse.
- If you feel something like a matchstick at your cervix, your IUCD has slipped and you should not rely on it for contraception until you see your Family Planning Doctor who may change the device.

How reliable is it?

- About 1 woman in every 100 who uses it will get pregnant each year.
- Some of the latest ones are even more effective.

Who's suitable to use the IUCD?

❖ Women in a stable relationship who don't want to use other forms of contraception for several years are the most suitable.

Who's NOT suitable to use the IUCD?

❖ It's not ideal for young women who haven't had children – although in some circumstances it can still be used.
❖ It isn't recommended if you have or have had:
1. a sexually transmitted infection or pelvic inflammatory disease *(PID)*.
2. heavy, irregular or painful vaginal bleeding without a known cause.
3. an ectopic *(tubal)* pregnancy.
4. you or your partner have sex with other people.
5. an allergy to copper.

My friend says that the coil/IUCD causes infection. Is this true?

❖ No, it is not true.
❖ The coil/IUCD is a sterile device.
❖ If you have an existing infection at your cervix at the time of insertion, that can be pushed into your uterus and cause pelvic infection (PID/pelvic inflammatory disease).

Will I be tested for anything before I have an IUCD fitted?

❖ Many clinics test for an infection called *chlamydia* before inserting an IUCD. Some suggest you're fully screened for infection, at a GUM clinic, beforehand.
❖ This is wise and helps to prevent pelvic infection, which could put your fertility at risk.

Are there any benefits from using it apart from preventing pregnancy?

❖ No, there aren't.

For how many years can I use it?

❖ You can use an IUCD for between 5-10+ years depending on the device used.
❖ If you want to become pregnant, you can ask for it to be removed earlier.

Do diarrhoea, vomiting or antibiotics affect it?

❖ No.

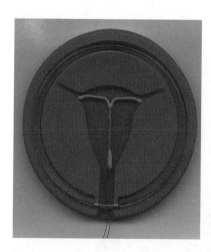

SEXplained...® © 1999 Helen Knox

Must I stop using it and let my body have a break?

❖ No, not unless you catch a sexually transmitted infection.

Will it control my periods?

❖ No, it won't.

Will it make my periods heavier or lighter?

❖ Modern IUCD's are smaller than their predecessors *(were used in the past)* and periods shouldn't be affected.
❖ They may last a little longer and compared with taking the Pill they'll be a little heavier. That's because the Pill makes periods lighter.

Left - coil correctly in uterus.
Below - coil slipping into cervical canal. May soon be felt at cervix when checking threads. Use extra protection and seek medical advice.

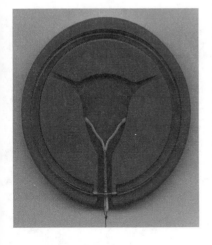

What should I be aware of if my girlfriend's using an IUCD?

❖ Her outward appearance doesn't change when she's using the IUCD, so it's up to you to help her check that it's still in place before you have sex. You can do this during foreplay by gently checking that you can feel the threads of the IUCD at her cervix.
❖ Diarrhoea, vomiting antibiotics or other drugs won't put either of you at increased risk of pregnancy.
❖ Remember: your girlfriend's not protected from sexually transmitted infections when using the IUCD on its own. So, if you're unfaithful to her, you could put her at risk if you don't use a condom. The only way to protect yourself fully from unplanned pregnancy AND infection is to use a condom during sex, *at all times*.

Do recreational drugs affect its reliability?

❖ No. Not as far as is known.
❖ Drugs can, however, be bad for your long-term physical and mental health and can increase your risk of contracting sexually transmitted infections.
❖ If you dehydrate you are more likely to get thrombosis *(blood clots)*.

Will the IUCD make me put on weight?

❖ No, it won't affect your weight.

Will it protect me from pregnancy AND infection?

❖ No, it won't protect you from infection. The only way is to use a condom.

Is it reversible?

❖ Yes, completely, upon removal.

When does it start to work?

❖ As soon as it's in place.

Do I have to have sex to use it?

❖ No, but there's no other reason for having one except for contraception.

Can I use it safely if I smoke?

❖ Yes.

Are there any disadvantages to using it?

❖ Yes. If you catch a sexually transmitted infection it can pass more easily into your womb than when other methods of contraception are used.

❖ Complications rarely occur from fitting but there is a small risk with IUCD's of having an ectopic *(tubal)* pregnancy.

Do I need to have a check-up after it's fitted?

❖ Yes, you should have a check-up after six weeks, and then every 6-12 months, to make sure that everything is OK.

Can I use tampons with an IUCD?

❖ Yes, you can use tampons but wait and use sanitary towels *(pads)* until after your first period in case the IUCD comes out with your first period.

❖ If you use tampons after your first period <u>always</u> check the thread(s) afterwards to make sure the IUCD hasn't come out during menstruation.

What is an IUS?

* IUS stands for Intra-Uterine System.
* An IUS is a contraceptive device, similar to a coil, with slow release hormone *(progestogen)* on it instead of the copper, used on an IUCD.
* It's called a *Mirena®*.

How does it work?

* It releases the hormone to the lining of your womb and alters its conditions to prevent you becoming pregnant.
* It thickens the mucus at your cervix, which prevents sperm entering your womb.
* It prevents some women from ovulating or releasing an egg, although most women still ovulate.

How reliable is it?

* Very reliable indeed.
* Almost 100% of pregnancies are prevented for users of the IUS.
* It's so good that it's commonly offered to prevent pregnancy instead of a sterilisation.

Who's suitable to use the IUS?

* It's suitable for women who've given birth. Others can have it inserted with or without local anaesthetic.

IUS

Can it be used for Emergency Contraception like the IUD?

* No, it should not be used as Emergency Contraception.

Who's NOT suitable to use the IUS?

* Women who are pregnant must not use it. Women who have or have had:
1. active liver infection or growth.
2. undiagnosed abnormal vaginal bleeding.
3. infection, or at risk of infection.
4. a history of heart or circulatory disease.

Are there any benefits from using it apart from preventing pregnancy?

* Yes, there are.
* It can help some women who get very heavy periods due to fibroids *(non-cancerous growths in the uterus)* but not all; depending on the fibroid.
* Periods are usually far less painful, lighter and shorter.

How is it fitted?

* An IUS is inserted under sterile conditions by a specially trained Family Planning Doctor – usually in the first week of your period.

When does it start to work?

* As soon as it's in place, provided it is fitted within 7 days of menstruation starting.

For how many years can I use it?

❖ It's licensed for 5 years' use. It can be removed sooner if you want to get pregnant.

Do diarrhoea, vomiting or antibiotics affect it?

❖ No.

Should I stop using an IUS and give my body a break?

❖ No.

Will it control my periods or make them heavier or lighter?

❖ No it won't control their timing but your periods will become lighter and less painful.

❖ You may experience irregular bleeding or spotting in the first few months of use.

What should I be aware of if my girlfriend's using an IUS?

❖ Her outward appearance doesn't change when she's using the IUS, so it's up to you to help her check that it's still in place before you have sex. You can do this during foreplay by gently checking that you can feel the threads of the IUS at her cervix.

❖ Diarrhoea, vomiting antibiotics or other drugs won't put either of you at increased risk of pregnancy.

❖ Remember: your girlfriend's not protected from sexually transmitted infections when using the IUS on its own. So, if you're unfaithful to her, you could put her at risk if you don't use a condom. The only way to protect yourself fully from unplanned pregnancy AND infection is to use a condom during sex, *at all times*.

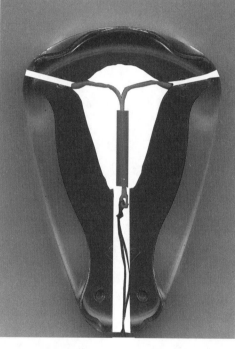

View of IUS in model uterus

Can I use tampons with an IUS?

❖ Yes, you can use tampons but wait and use sanitary towels *(pads)* until after your first period in case the IUS comes out with your first period.

❖ If you use tampons after your first period <u>always</u> check the thread(s) afterwards to make sure the IUS hasn't come out during menstruation.

Do recreational drugs affect its reliability?

❖ No. Not as far as is known.

❖ Drugs can, however, be bad for your long-term physical and mental health and can increase your risk of contracting sexually transmitted infections.

❖ If you dehydrate you are more likely to get thrombosis *(blood clots)*.

Will the IUS make me put on weight?

❖ No, not as far as is known.

Will it protect me from pregnancy AND infection?

❖ No, it won't protect you from infection. The only way is to use a condom.

Is it reversible?

❖ Yes, completely, upon removal.

Do I have to have sex to use it?

❖ No – *see benefits on page 85.*

Can I use it safely if I smoke?

❖ Yes.

Safer sex saves your life.

Hickey Etienne
Youth Worker,
south London

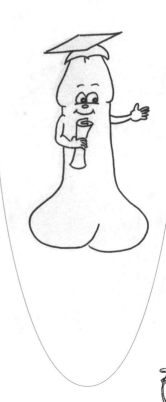

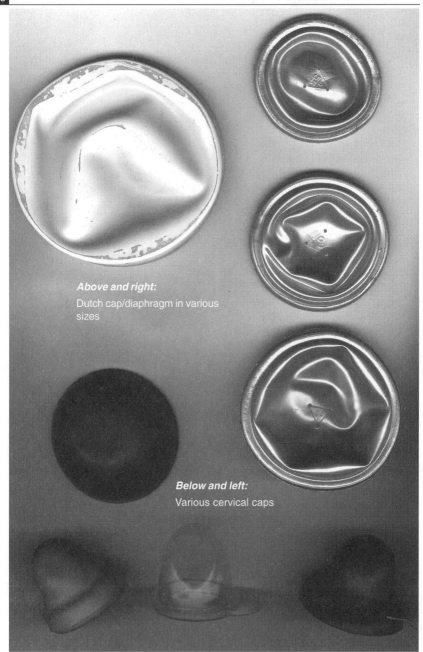

Above and right:
Dutch cap/diaphragm in various sizes

Below and left:
Various cervical caps

Selection of contraceptive caps

What is the Cap?

- The Cap is a latex or rubber dome which fits over your cervix.
- There are different varieties – eg. the Dutch cap or diaphragm, Dumas vault cap, Prentif cavity rim cervical cap and the Vimule.
- The *Honey Cap* is available; but this is not given free at Family Planning Clinics, is extremely expensive and is not generally recommended.
- The Oves® cervical cap is new. It is disposable and is made of silicone. It's suitable for some women who get recurrent cystitis. It's not available on the NHS, but can be purchased from the chemist.

How does it work?

- It forms a barrier between your eggs and your partner's sperm, thereby preventing pregnancy.

How reliable is it?

- It's not as reliable as the injection, the IUS, sterilisation, the Pill, mini-pill *(POP)*, the IUCD or the male condom.
- But, if you're extremely organised and good about using it correctly, every single time you have sex, it can be a good method and can be over 90% effective.
- It's more reliable if you put strips of spermicidal cream or jel *(jelly)* on both sides of the cap, before insertion.
- It may be more effective if you wait until you are in your mid 20's to 40's; or in a long-term, stable relationship.

Who's suitable to use it?

- It's suitable for women for whom a pregnancy would not be disastrous.
- Women who can't use, or don't want to use, any other method of contraception.
- For women who are very organised and for whom sex needs to be planned not spontaneous *(as with the Pill)*.

Who's NOT suitable to use it?

- It's not suitable for women who get recurrent, common cystitis *(bladder inflammation)*.
- Women who really don't want to be pregnant.

Are there any non-contra-ceptive benefits?

- Some women use it to contain the menstrual flow and protect their bedding, if they have sex during their period.

How do I use it?

- Because vaginas come in different shapes and sizes a cap must be fitted individually by a Family Planning trained Nurse or Doctor.
- You'll be given a *practise cap*, shown how to use it and allowed to take it home for a week, to practise inserting and removing it on your own.
- Even when practising your insertion technique, you should add spermicidal cream or jel, before inserting the cap.
- You shouldn't rely upon it as a method of contraception in that time because the *practise cap* may have a hole in it.

Why would a practice cap have holes in it?

❖ Holes prevent you from using the cap for contraception until the Nurse or Doctor says you've inserted and removed it correctly.

❖ This gives you time to learn the correct technique of insertion, how to check that it's in the correct position and also to give your partner the opportunity to become familiar with this method of contraception.

❖ Once you've mastered the technique, you'll be given your own, new cap, without holes.

What if I want to have sex in my practise time?

❖ If you want to have sex during practise either use a condom or other reliable method of birth control. You can leave your practice cap in place to see how sex feels when it's in place.

Will sex feel different with a cap?

❖ No. Fitted correctly, you won't be aware that you're wearing a cap when you're having sex.

❖ If it's not the right size, nor positioned correctly, you MAY or may not notice a strange sensation.

Will my partner feel it during sex?

❖ No, he shouldn't feel a correctly fitted cap during sex.

❖ Sometimes, the man notices a slight stinging sensation from the spermicide, if he's not using a condom. If he notices this, change spermicide.

How long must I have it in, before I have sex?

❖ You can insert it any time up to 3 hours before you have sex.

❖ If you exceed *(go over)* this time before having sex, simply put more spermicide into your vagina – or remove, wash and re-insert your cap.

❖ Spermicide in the form of a pessary – solid spermicide which melts at body temperature; or via an applicator – like a syringe without a needle; may be used.

Can I take the cap out straight after I have sex?

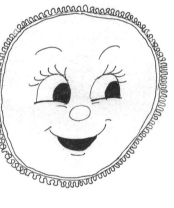

❖ No, you can't because of the risk of pregnancy.

❖ After sex you must leave the cap in place for 6 hours for the spermicide to kill any ejaculated sperm, otherwise you'll just stun them.

What if we want to have sex again within 6 hours?

❖ If you have sex again in those 6 hours, you should leave the cap in place AND insert more spermicide into your vagina. Start counting your 6 hours again, from the second time after you had sex.

The Cap

How long can I leave the cap in for and keep *topping up* the spermicide?

❖ Try not to keep it in for any longer than 30 hours because of the risk of developing Toxic Shock Syndrome.

❖ *For further information on TSS see page 46.*

How do I take the cap out and what must I do with it?

❖ To take out your cap, simply wash your hand, insert a finger into your vagina, hook the edge of your cap and pull it out.

❖ When you've removed it, just wash it under running water and pat it dry with a towel before replacing it in its carrying box.

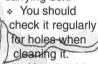

❖ You should check it regularly for holes when cleaning it.

❖ You should be shown how to look after your cap when you're taught how to use it by the Family Planning Nurse.

For how many years can I use it?

❖ Caps usually have a life span of 12-24 months' use.

❖ However, should you develop a vaginal infection, you should ask for a new cap, to prevent reinfection.

Can anything damage the cap?

❖ Some vaginal medication is oil-based, which can rot the latex of the cap (and condom), so you should avoid sex altogether when being treated.

❖ If in doubt, always ask your local Pharmacist or your condom supplier for advice.

❖ *For further information, turn to the list of lubricants and vaginal medication on page 154-155.*

When doesn't the cap work?

You risk pregnancy:

❖ when it's inserted wrongly ie. if you don't have your cervix covered.

❖ if you don't use it every time you have sex.

❖ if you use it without spermicide it's much less reliable.

❖ if you take it out before the 6 hours are up, after sex.

❖ if you fail to *top-up* with more spermicide and have sex again within your 6 waiting hours.

Is it affected by diarrhoea, vomiting or antibiotics?

❖ No, but it can be affected by some vaginal oil-based medication.

Will it control my periods?

❖ No, it won't.

❖ If you have your cap in when your period starts, your blood loss will collect inside your cap.

Will it make my periods heavier or lighter?

❖ It won't affect your periods.

SEXplained...® © 1999 Helen Knox

What should I be aware of if my girlfriend's using a cap?

❖ You should know how it should feel when it's in her vagina correctly.

❖ You should check, during foreplay, that the latex of the cap covers her cervix.

❖ You will find her cervix approximatley a fingers depth inside her vagina. It feels like a round hard lump with a dimple in the centre - similar to the end of your nose.

❖ If you don't think it's covered, don't enter.

❖ At the fertile time of her cycle, you might feel safer if you use a condom, for extra protection against pregnancy.

❖ Using a condom routinely with the cap would, though, greatly increase the success rate of this method of contraception.

Do recreational drugs affect its reliability?

❖ No, they don't.

❖ Drugs can, however, be bad for your long-term physical and mental health and can increase your risk of contracting sexually transmitted infections.

❖ If you dehydrate you are more likely to get thrombosis *(blood clots)*.

Will it make me put on weight?

❖ No, but if you lose or gain 7lbs or more, you should return to your clinic and have your cap checked for the correct fit.

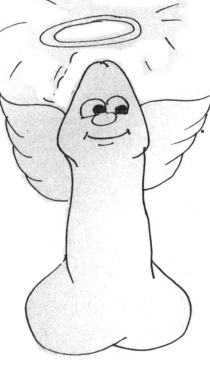

Will it protect me from pregnancy AND infection?

❖ You gain some protection to your cervix but it doesn't prevent transmission of infection.

❖ In the laboratory spermicide has been found to kill some germs but unless a condom is used, your vaginal surface area is still at risk of infection, as is your external genital area.

❖ Using a condom AND a cap gives better protection against both pregnancy and infection.

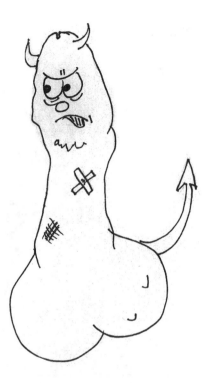

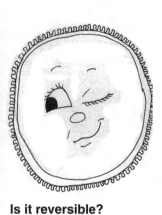

Is it reversible?

❖ Yes. As soon as it's removed or; if it's inserted incorrectly, you're at risk of pregnancy.

When does it start to work?

❖ It's effective as soon as it's in the correct position.

Can I use it safely if I smoke?

❖ Yes, you can.

Do I have to have a check-up after I am fitted with my cap?

❖ Yes, you should return a week after fitting, to see that you're able to use it correctly and get a new cap.

❖ Thereafter, you should have a check-up every 6 months – unless you lose or gain 7lbs or more in weight. In that case, you should return earlier for a check-up.

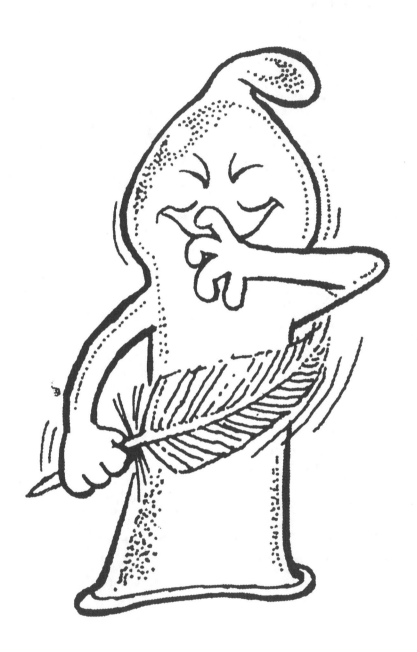

Contraceptive implants

❖ Contraceptive implants are another method of female contraception consisting of small rods containing the hormone, progestogen.

❖ They're inserted under the skin of your upper arm and slowly release the hormone into your body for various lengths of time, depending upon the implant used.

The Male Pill

❖ Much research is under way to develop and market a male pill. However, male fertility is harder to control, since men produce millions of sperm all the time.

❖ Trials have shown that it *is* possible to control sperm production, but unwanted side effects of the drug combinations must be overcome. Therefore this method is still some years away from common use.

❖ Although it may be a good idea for men who are well motivated to use it, surveys have shown that many women would be reluctant to trust a man who says he's taken his pill – in case he hasn't and was just saying he had – to get her to agree to his sexual advances!

❖ When, eventually, the male pill becomes widely available, it will only give protection against pregnancy. It won't give any protection against sexually transmitted infection.

Natural Family Planning (NFP)

❖ NFP is also known as using the *safe time* but it isn't the first method of choice for young women whose bodies are growing and adjusting; or those who have some medical condition such as Polycystic Ovary Syndrome (PCOS), etc. **See also Persona®.**

❖ NFP requires close observation of all your body signs and symptoms over 6-12 months, which you are taught by a specially trained NFP teacher.

❖ The menstrual cycle can be complicated to understand and several things can mislead your observations.

❖ Long periods of abstinence *(no sex)* are required if you're relying on this method as your sole protection.

❖ Your partner should also understand it fully because there are lots of times when you can't have unprotected sex and they're mostly the times when you feel more randy or sexy!

Persona®

- ❖ This is an electronic computerised device, which can be bought at a pharmacy.
- ❖ It analyses specimens of your urine and works out whether you're at the fertile time of your cycle and at risk of pregnancy if you have regular menstrual cycles between 23 and 35 days in length.
- ❖ It's easy to use but not suitable for all women, especially young women whose bodies are still developing or women who have an irregular menstrual cycle.
- ❖ It's not recommended for women who are breast feeding, using hormonal medication, have liver or kidney disease, menopausal symptoms or the gynaecological condition called Polycystic Ovary Syndrome *(PCOS)*.
- ❖ It's not recommended for women taking the antibiotic *tetracycline*.
- ❖ It gives no protection against HIV or other sexually transmitted infections.
- ❖ There are no side effects but you must follow the instructions carefully.
- ❖ It's an alternative method of Natural Family Planning.

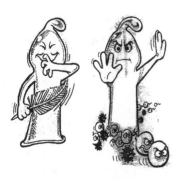

Sterilisation

- ❖ Sterilisation should be considered permanent surgical intervention to prevent pregnancy.
- ❖ In men, the *vas deferens* and in women the *fallopian tubes* are cut, to prevent sperm or eggs from meeting.
- ❖ Male sterilisation *(vasectomy)* is easy, quick and effective when you've decided you don't want any risk of pregnancy – or have completed your family.
- ❖ Female sterilisation involves slightly more complicated surgery. Many gynaecologists now recommend the Mirena® *(the IUS)* while you wait for surgery, as it's so reliable. Many women decide to keep their Mirena® instead of having surgical sterilisation.
- ❖ The choice is yours, but you should know that any surgery carries a risk and no method of contraception including sterilisation *(except no sex/ celibacy)* can guarantee 100% protection against pregnancy.

Vaginal rings, contraceptive vaccines, contraceptive patches and other possibilities

- ❖ There are several methods of contraception under development. Most, however, are some years away from being in general use.

Contraceptive Word Search

C	O	M	B	I	N	E	D	O	R	A	L	S	F	V	P	A	D	G
O	C	Z	P	G	A	S	E	A	E	O	U	Y	A	Z	L	P	I	P
N	B	L	A	F	T	R	V	I	C	Q	B	S	M	T	A	H	B	M
T	D	R	P	L	U	T	I	N	J	E	C	T	I	O	N	E	J	K
R	V	T	A	M	R	S	C	O	C	A	T	E	L	T	N	O	N	E
A	L	F	V	M	A	L	E	A	A	T	E	M	Y	H	I	V	I	R
C	O	I	L	U	L	G	C	X	R	O	M	A	N	C	N	B	U	T
E	M	E	R	G	E	N	C	Y	G	E	J	C	E	H	G	F	M	A
P	O	P	S	T	E	R	I	L	I	S	A	T	I	O	N	B	D	F
T	H	E	C	A	P	A	C	O	N	D	O	M	C	R	U	M	B	A
I	N	T	R	A	U	T	E	R	I	N	E	S	Y	S	T	E	M	S
V	C	E	L	I	B	A	C	Y	U	M	T	Y	N	R	E	T	R	O
E	F	E	M	A	L	E	Y	O	D	I	A	P	H	R	A	G	M	G
P	R	O	G	E	S	T	O	G	E	N	O	N	L	Y	P	I	L	L
I	M	P	L	A	N	T	P	A	T	C	H	T	I	C	R	U	E	S
L	T	I	T	C	H	P	S	F	R	A	B	R	L	O	M	S	T	A
L	O	V	E	R	S	Y	S	E	X	P	L	A	I	N	E	D	H	K

- ❖ combined oral
- ❖ contraceptive pill
- ❖ the cap
- ❖ intrauterine
- ❖ injection
- ❖ system * 2
- ❖ device
- ❖ COC
- ❖ POP
- ❖ IUD
- ❖ IUS
- ❖ progestogen only pill
- ❖ implant
- ❖ diaphragm
- ❖ natural
- ❖ family
- ❖ planning
- ❖ sterilisation
- ❖ condom

- ❖ emergency
- ❖ patch
- ❖ female
- ❖ male
- ❖ no
- ❖ celibacy
- ❖ lover
- ❖ SEXplained
- ❖ coil
- ❖ pad
- ❖ titch

For answers: see page 181

SEXplained...® © 1999 Helen Knox

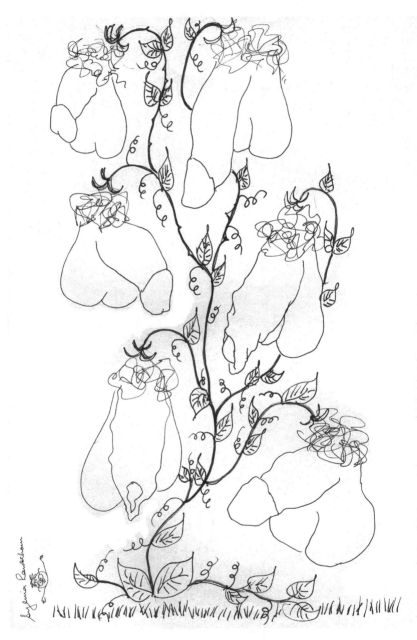

Willius Floppius Variegata.
The Willy plant.

Sex is never compulsory. You should never do anything just to please someone, particularly if you feel uncomfortable or because of peer pressure.

I thought sex meant male or female, so why do people say they have sex?

❖ It's short for have sexual intercourse.

Why do people have sex?

People have sex because:

❖ it makes you feel nice.
❖ to have babies.
❖ to feel close to another person.
❖ to feel loved for a short while.
❖ to get a cuddle.
❖ sometimes they feel pressure from friends that they should *do it*.
❖ some people have sex to make money.

Why do people have sex if they want a cuddle?

❖ Some people find it hard to admit they simply want a cuddle, so they use having sex as a way to feel physically close to another person.
❖ Others fear being rejected by their partner if they say they don't want to have sex, so carry on in the hope of getting their cuddle afterwards.

If someone wants to have sex with me, does it mean they love me?

❖ Not necessarily.
❖ It may be lust or just physical attraction.

❖ If you've taken time to get to know each other well, you'll probably feel closer and may even feel as if you're in love.

My partner says that if I love him/her I'd have sex with him/her. S/he just doesn't understand that I'm not ready to have sex. Why do they do this and what should I do?

❖ Tell them to grow up.
❖ This statement is old as time itself! It's a trick and usually backfires on whoever tells you such rubbish. It's unfair emotional pressure which aims to get you to give in.
❖ If you feel you don't want sex – listen to your heart.
❖ You always have the right to say NO.
❖ Don't have sex with anyone until you're ready and are sure YOU want to do it.
❖ It's easy to confuse having sex with being in love. Don't let anyone make you feel bad about your decision not to have sex.
❖ It doesn't mean you don't care for your partner – just that you're not ready for – or don't want this type of relationship yet.
❖ If s/he really cares about you they'll stop pestering you and stay friends.
❖ If they don't stop they're silly and will risk you going right off them. A nicer person's probably waiting round the corner!
❖ *Remember: there are plenty more fish in the sea!*

SEXplained...® © 1999 Helen Knox

Growing Up and New Experiences

My boyfriend says he'll leave me if I don't do what he wants.

❖ Some boyfriend! Let him leave, if that's his attitude towards you!

❖ If you give in to his unfair, immature bullying he'll only try another way to get his own way.

❖ However nice, good looking, charming, sexy or anything else that he may be when he wants something, he's trying to coerce *(manipulate)* you into doing something against your will.

❖ If he doesn't change his tune, he'll probably lose you anyway with such a childish attitude.

❖ He doesn't sound worthy of your affection. This sort of attitude is more likely to be a complete turn off to you, anyway.

❖ Don't fall for his sweet talk. It's designed to get your clothing off. He's just shown you that he doesn't really care about how you feel, so do you really need someone like this in your life?

How do young men masturbate?

❖ If you stroke the sensitive area at the head of your penis and think of something sexy, you'll probably have an erection.

❖ Make a fist around the shaft of your penis and move this up and down its length – slowly, at first but faster as the pleasurable feelings increase and you near orgasm.

❖ After ejaculation your penis goes soft *(flaccid)* as you relax.

❖ As you explore your body more, and with practice, you'll develop your own masturbation technique.

❖ Like women, you may get pleasure from massaging areas of your body called erogenous zones – eg. your nipples or another area you find sensitive and pleasurable.

How do young women masturbate?

❖ When you're sexually aroused – either by thought or sensation – your vagina produces a welcoming fluid *(lubricant)* to make insertion of a penis more comfortable.

❖ Your clitoris is extremely sensitive and when rubbed gently it enlarges and erects.

❖ Gently massaging or rubbing it can feel very nice and gradually give you intense pleasure.

❖ You might also use a finger from your other hand to copy the movement a penis makes during sex – moving in and out of your vagina, gently.

❖ Some women use sex toys such as vibrators, dildo's or similar shaped objects to mimic the size or shape of a penis instead of their finger.

❖ Masturbation is similar to the heavy petting of foreplay performed by your partner.

❖ As with men, you may get pleasure from massaging areas of your body called erotic zones such eg. your nipples or another area you find sensitive and pleasurable.

What does having an orgasm feel like?

Different people feel different strengths of sensation.

For both man and women

❖ The largest part of sex is in your mind and your body reacts physically to its stimulation.

❖ Orgasm doesn't happen, auto-matically, every time you have sex especially if you try too hard for one or if you're not really in the mood.

❖ Some people get terribly upset and feel it's the man's duty to give a woman her orgasm. This isn't true.

❖ Orgasm is more likely to happen when you're totally relaxed. It may be because you want purely physical sex or because you're *making love* together.

❖ With some practice, you can think yourself into and out of orgasm mode, control it and decide when you want to *come/cum*.

❖ You'll breathe more rapidly. Your pulse and heart rate will rise.

❖ You may feel a warm glow throughout your body and sweat slightly before breaking out in a rash *(sex flush)* after you reach orgasm.

For young men

❖ It's more obvious than for young women, because you ejaculate. This gives you intense pleasure as the semen and sperm are forced out of your penis by muscular contractions.

❖ After ejaculation your penis softens as you relax.

For young women

❖ The centre for orgasm is your clitoris, which swells during sexual arousal *(just like a penis)* and your vagina, which produces a lubricant so that a penis can slip in and out easily.

❖ There's a gradual build up of pleasurable sensation, your breathing becomes deeper and more rapid, your heart beats faster and your vagina may go into involuntary spasm as you reach orgasm, with your body becoming tense all over.

❖ After orgasm it relaxes and you feel a warm glow throughout your body and you may notice a rash *(sex flush)* all over.

It's so complicated!

❖ Yes, it is complicated. That's why taking time to get to know someone well, and talking openly about what you both want or don't want, is the best way to understand what's happening.

❖ Today, virginity, monogamy *(staying with only one sexual partner)* and celibacy *(not having sex)* are actually quite trendy.

❖ Along with the temporary physical pleasure from sex, there can be considerable emotional pain.

❖ It's better to wait until you're more mature and in a stable/settled friendship before starting a sexual relationship.

❖ Once you give away your virginity you can't get it back.

❖ Also, for young women, sex before you're physically mature *(approx. 23 years of age)* can increase the risk of damage to your cervix – especially if you smoke cigarettes and/or have sex with someone who's had a sexually transmitted infection.

❖ Furthermore, you risk infertility or difficulty getting pregnant if you catch *gonorrhoea* or *chlamydia* and don't get it treated quickly.

❖ Many books are available about sex, which you could read with your partner when you feel ready to learn more about the subject.

What's heavy petting/foreplay?

For both sexes

❖ First, always be clear about how far you are prepared to go and what you're prepared to allow. If you change your mind, and don't want to go further with foreplay, make your wishes clear. Try to do this without hurting your partner's feelings to enable their arousal to subside.

❖ There are generally two types of foreplay.

1– Psychological foreplay *(in your mind)* – eg. talking seductively to each other, dressing in a particular fashion *(sexy under-wear)*, watching films together or listening to soft music to set the mood or scene – and lots more.

2– Physical foreplay *(play before sex)* is similar to masturbation and usually takes place before or perhaps instead of penetration.

❖ You may go as far as reaching orgasm *(climax/coming)* during foreplay, but penetration doesn't take place at this stage.

❖ Women can sometimes have multiple orgasms; men usually ejaculate only once then need a

bit of a rest before starting again.

❖ Some men can control them-selves very well, delay orgasm and make sex last a long time.

❖ Other men aren't able to control themselves very well and reach orgasm within minutes *(or seconds)* of penetration.

For young women

❖ Generally you'll get physically turned on *(aroused)* when your breasts or your clitoris are gently rubbed or massaged.

❖ Clitoral arousal, in particular, stimulates your vagina to make a lubricant or *welcoming fluid*.

❖ You may then allow your partner to go a bit further, to the stage commonly called *fingering*.

❖ This is when they gently insert one or two fingers into your vagina to simulate the movement a penis makes during sex.

❖ At the same time, they continue to rub your clitoris gently.

❖ Before long, if you're relaxed, you'll start to have an orgasm.

❖ You may, however, reach orgasm without any finger penetration but from breast or clitoral stimulation, alone.

❖ With some practice, you'll be able to learn to control your orgasm – ie. to have it as and when you decide. But, if you're not relaxed or feeling safe, you're unlikely to reach orgasm.

❖ If you're unable to masturbate to orgasm and are worried about it, your GP or Family Planning Clinic can advise you.

For young men

❖ This is when your partner masturbates your penis with their hand. *(Commonly known as a hand job, wank or hand relief.)*

❖ They gently squeeze and massage along the shaft and/or tip of your penis which, when you're relaxed, stimulates and gives pleasure.

❖ If you're unable to masturbate to orgasm on your own and are worried about it, your GP or Family Planning Clinic can advise you or refer you if you would like help.

Some people say that boys want sex but girls want to make love. What's the difference and why?

❖ To many people, making love sounds more emotionally involved, it's usually more planned, slower and more tender.

❖ Having sex is generally considered to be just a physical thing – relatively quick and without much emotion.

❖ Men *and* women can have sex without any emotions becoming involved; so, it's not just a male thing.

How soon should we have sex?

❖ It's becoming trendy to be able to say you're still a virgin, so there's no rush at all to start having sex.

❖ It's best to wait until you're both absolutely sure that the time is right and until you're safely protected from the risk of unplanned pregnancy and/or infection. You have the rest of your life to enjoy it.

❖ Sometimes you might not want to do something but feel you should go along with your partner out of fear of rejection if you don't agree.

❖ Communication is the key, so talk to each other to see what you both like, want to do, or don't want to do.

❖ Don't be scared to speak out. You are probably just as nervous as each other.

❖ There's really no rush to have sex.

❖ You'll need practise if you use condoms. The *Double Dutch* method is widely advised these days – ie. being on the Pill *(or other contraceptive method)* AND using condoms, even if you're both virgins.

Sex is an ultimate connection between two people and as such should not be hurried or forced.
You alone know when you are truely ready, so don't allow anyone to bully or coerce you.
Sex will always be better when you are mentally and physically prepared.

Felicity Ethnic
Comedian

What about sex outside marriage?

❖ Many cultures and religions still frown upon sex outside marriage. However, millions of people the world over are sexually active without being married *(fornicate)*.

❖ No one can dictate how you live your life once you reach the legal age of consent.

❖ It's your choice whether you wait until marriage or have sex outside it.

❖ Many people don't want to marry but choose to stay in long-term committed and faithful relationships, for a variety of reasons.

❖ Being made to feel guilty for having sex without being married can cause long-term psychological problems for some people.

❖ The desire to have sex is an animal instinct and it's not helpful to damn others for their choice or circumstances.

❖ Sexual abuse, rape or sexual assault outside or within marriage is an entirely different matter. They're illegal and frowned upon by most religions or cultures around the world – some to a greater extent than others.

❖ If you're married and have sex outside it *(commit adultery)*, that's a matter for your conscience. It can, however, lead to numerous emotional, financial, legal or physical problems. This may include pregnancy and/or sexually transmitted infection.

❖ Unless you're forced to have sex, the choice is yours and yours alone.

My boyfriend says he *needs* to have sex with me

❖ This is selfish rubbish and typical emotional pressure to make you give in.

❖ He doesn't **need** to have sex, he **wants** to have sex.

❖ He won't die if you don't give in to him, whatever he says or thinks!

❖ He can always relieve himself by masturbation!

❖ It won't make him blind, deaf or dumb. His penis belongs to him, so he'll come to no harm if he masturbates instead.

❖ Let him sulk, if he's that childish – but don't give in unless YOU want to have sex, too, and you are safely protected from pregnancy AND infection.

If you're ignorant about all contraception, then you're no better than the others you see around.

Be better than the rest.

Kat
Choreographer
& All Round Entertainer

I'm still a virgin but all the other kids at school boast about how many times they've had sex and how many partners they've had. I feel left out, should I find someone and just *do it*?

❖ No, you shouldn't just *do it*.

❖ They may be making it up!

❖ Today, it seems more sensible to be able to boast about still being a virgin!

❖ Studies show that the majority of young women who choose to have sex early, regret it later and wish they'd waited until they were older.

❖ A lot of young men also wish they'd waited until they were older.

❖ Let sex happen when it feels right for *you* and you're *sure* it's what you want.

❖ Having sex is not *always* what it's cracked up to be, so don't panic and do it just to tell your friends you've done it.

❖ Sex can be lovely when it's *part* of a caring, loving relationship but it's only part of any relationship.

❖ Being good pals with your partner is more important in the long run.

Keep God in your heart.
Keep your focus.
Remember your purpose
on the planet.

Roger Wright
Lead singer
True Identity

What does French kissing mean?

❖ French kissing is when, during lip to lip kissing, your partner slips their tongue into your mouth and feels your tongue.

❖ They may suck your tongue gently and you can suck theirs.

❖ It's also known as deep or wet kissing.

❖ You don't have to be in France or kissing a French person to French kiss!

I think I love someone, they're gorgeous, then it goes and I fancy someone else. Sometimes I fancy two people at once. Is this common?

❖ Yes, it's very common and it's all part of growing up.

❖ These fleeting feelings are usually called a *crush*.

❖ You'll probably find you experience these same feelings again as you get older.

Do erect nipples mean we want sex?

❖ They could mean you're sexually aroused – there again, you could be cold!

❖ The cold makes the muscles around your nipples contract *(shorten)* so they're more obvious.

❖ By the way, this happens to men *and* women.

Growing Up and New Experiences

I don't know what to do with my partner, so how do I become *the best at sex*?

❖ There's no such thing as becoming the best at sex. Each person has his or her own opinion of what good sex is and their own technique.

❖ It's most important to be able to talk to each other; and to listen to what your partner says they'd like to do or would like you to do.

❖ You should then be honest with each other, not just go along with what they say they'd like, for two reasons:

(a) they may not really want to do it but think you want them to try or ask.

(b) you should never let anyone persuade you to do or try anything, just to keep him/her happy and not yourself.

❖ It can take a lot of time, patience, understanding, practice and romance – plus a lot of genuine care, to improve your skill as a lover.

❖ Always treat your partner with respect and as you'd like to be treated.

❖ Sometimes, being honest with yourself, and then someone else, about sex is quite difficult but it's the best way forward.

I've heard boys talking about a *fanny fart*. What's that?

❖ Since there's only one entrance/ exit to your vagina, air can get trapped in it when you have sex in certain positions.

❖ This sometimes escapes noisily – but it doesn't smell!

❖ It's common and harmless.

Does or should sex hurt a woman?

❖ No, sex between two consenting partners shouldn't hurt.

❖ During foreplay and sex you should be gentle and not appear in an obvious hurry.

❖ Listen to what your partner wants.

❖ It's usually wise to spend the length of time they want on foreplay, so that they can relax and get in the mood, rather than just spend a minute or two and think *that's long enough*! Nobody would thank you for that!

❖ If you're in a hurry or pressure your female partner into having sex, there won't be sufficient time for her body to make the special *welcoming fluid* in her vagina for your penis to slip in easily.

❖ If she's dry or tense, sex is likely to be uncomfortable for both of you.

❖ If there's pain during sex, you should stop.

❖ If your partner wants you to continue you may find that a different position may help. Some sexually transmitted infections cause pain during sex.

❖ If the problem is not from dryness or from the position you're in, visit your Family Planning Clinic, GUM/STI Clinic or your GP for advice.

❖ Sex will, however, hurt women who have been circumcised, who are raped or anyone who is forced to have anal sex *(buggered/ sodomised)*. This is not sex between two caring and consenting partners.

❖ Never force yourself on anyone.

❖ If you're told to stop, then you **must** stop; otherwise you'll be committing a criminal offence.

❖ *For information see page 121.*

Do love-bites hurt and can they cause disease or harm?

* ❖ Love-bites can be uncomfortable.
* ❖ They cause bruising when blood is drawn to the surface levels underneath your skin by the pressure of sucking required to produce them.
* ❖ They cause embarrassment rather than any real harm or disease and they can look unattractive, especially when they begin to wear off.
* ❖ *Tip – Smearing toothpaste over them can sometimes help love-bites wear off a bit quicker!*

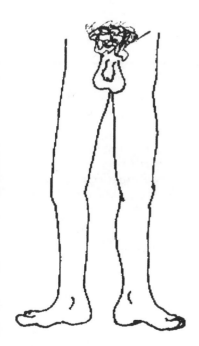

Why do I just want to have sex without any commitment?

* ❖ There could be many reasons why you don't want commitment.
* ❖ Only you know the answer but being honest with yourself may be quite difficult.
* ❖ If you tell the person with whom you're having sex how you feel before you just use them, you may find they feel the same way.
* ❖ You may be young and don't want to tie yourself down yet.
* ❖ You may be older and have been through a traumatic emotional experience. Therefore don't want to allow someone else to get to know you well enough to get hurt again.
* ❖ Perhaps you enjoy the chase and conquest rather than ongoing relationships.
* ❖ You may be scared to risk being let down by another person. Therefore, hold yourself back from loving and being loved in return.
* ❖ Perhaps you're scared of someone being dependent upon you and don't want that kind of responsibility.
* ❖ Always be honest rather than lead someone else on.
* ❖ If you know another reason and want help to resolve *(sort out)* your feelings but don't know where to start, contact your GP or Family Planning Clinic.

Why didn't my partner want to know me, after we had sex?

- ❖ Unfortunately this is quite common and may be due to several reasons.
- ❖ Wanting to have sex is an animal instinct.
- ❖ People don't always plan this, but it's commonly known as a *one-night stand*.
- ❖ Sometimes people simply want casual sex. Many people don't realise until afterwards that all the *sweet talk* has been used to make them feel wanted and desirable enough to agree.
- ❖ Even when you've known each other for a while, your emotions can change after you've had sex.
- ❖ These are not just a male thing. Women can want casual sex without any further commitment, too. It could be for the better – or for the worse!

- ❖ Sometimes the chase seems more exciting than catching your partner!
- ❖ Sex often gets better the more time you spend together, as your relationship gets stronger, and as your care and respect for each other grows into a loving relationship.
- ❖ That's a good reason to wait.

Is sex addictive?

- ❖ For some people it can become addictive.
- ❖ Sex between two consenting partners improves with time, and becomes a deeply satisfying part of their lives.
- ❖ Some people, however, do feel they're obsessed with sex.
- ❖ If you feel this way, ask your GP or Family Planning Clinic to refer you to a specialist in psycho-sexual medicine.

Do nothing in haste.

Do you cherish your life?
Do you look forward to tomorrow?
Is your life filled with brightness? No dwelling on past sorrow?
Can you truely say, your smiles come from within?
Are you happy enough to say a good day will begin?
Are you walking without a heavy and worried mind?
Can you happily say you can leave your past behind?
Were those special words said? Did you choose to believe?
Did you question the actions? Could you have been deceived?
Did you think for one moment, that your actions were rushed?
And in that one moment, so much could be sussed.
Had YOU taken the time, to make sure you were safe?
Think, before you walk.

Do nothing in haste!

Sheila Daley
Poet, London

Can I really get pregnant *before* my first period?

❖ Yes you can. *See page 23.*

Can I get pregnant if my boyfriend kisses me?

❖ No, kissing can't make you pregnant.

Do I have to have sex to get pregnant?

❖ No, it's possible to get pregnant without having sex.

❖ A virgin can get pregnant and remain, technically, a virgin.

❖ Expensive fertility treatments, surgery etc. are not the only ways to get pregnant without having sex!

How can I get pregnant without having sex, then?

❖ Pregnancy can occur without sexual intercourse occurring because the ejaculation of sperm is not always necessary to create a pregnancy. Many people – *adults included* – get this fact wrong!

❖ When a young man gets an erection there are about 3,000,000 sperm in the drop of clear fluid which appears at the tip of his penis.

❖ That's enough sperm to populate the whole of the Central American country of Honduras!

❖ If he just rubs his erection around the entrance to your vagina *(without putting it inside you)*, sperm could get into the fertile mucus you make before ovulation *(egg release)* and travel up to your fallopian tubes.

❖ If they meet an egg, *hey presto*, one unplanned pregnancy!

If I'm a virgin can I get pregnant like this?

❖ Yes, you can.

Can I get pregnant the first time I have sex?

❖ Yes, you can and many girls do.

❖ There's about a 1 in 3 chance of pregnancy each time you have unprotected sex at the fertile time of the month.

❖ You MAY get away with it, but many don't.

Can I get pregnant without having an orgasm?

❖ Yes, you can.

❖ Orgasm and fertility are unrelated.

❖ Orgasm has nothing to do with egg release.

Can I get pregnant standing up?

❖ Yes and many women have become pregnant in this position.

❖ The position in which you have sex makes no difference whatsoever.

❖ As long as sperm get into your fertile mucus *(the special fluid you make before egg release)* there's a chance of pregnancy.

Can I get pregnant by heavy petting or fingering?

❖ Generally, no.

❖ Not unless there are sperm on the fingers which get into your fertile mucus.

My friend uses heroin and her periods have stopped. Can she still get pregnant?

❖ Yes, she is still at risk of pregnancy if she has unprotected sex.

❖ Even though she hasn't got regular periods, it doesn't mean she isn't ovulating.

❖ She must use *Double Dutch* protection – ie. use a condom AND other reliable method of birth control – at all times.

❖ Her risk of contracting hepatitis and/or HIV is FAR greater than a non-drug user – *particularly* if she injects the heroin.

❖ *For further information on contraception see pages 49-97.*

When can I have a pregnancy test?

❖ A test cannot tell if you may become pregnant the day after unprotected sex or even the next week since it takes 5 days for a fertilised egg to implant. It's only after implantation that the hormone a pregnancy test detects starts to show in your urine *(HCG/ human chorionic gonadotrophin).*

❖ Therefore, you will have to wait at least a couple of weeks after unprotected sex until there is enough to detect.

Generally, you can have a pregnancy test

(a) If you miss a period after having sex, whether you were using contraception including condoms or were not using contraception or protection.

(b) If you have a light period after having sex.

(c) If you have a light period after taking Emergency Contraception.

(d) If you have a light period after an abortion or miscarriage.

(e) If you're using the combined Pill and not getting withdrawal bleeds *(periods).*

(f) To put your mind at rest if you're worried for another reason.

Where can I have a pregnancy test?

❖ If you take a specimen of your urine to a Family Planning Clinic or Brook Advisory Centre, they will test it and give you the result immediately.

❖ Your GP can send a sample of your urine to the laboratory. In this case you have to wait for the result.

❖ You can buy a home pregnancy testing kit at a pharmacy and do your own test.

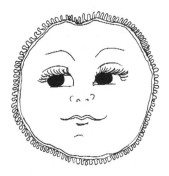

What if I find out I'm pregnant and don't know what to do or where to turn for help.

❖ Your GP or Family Planning Clinic can help or refer you for advice on antenatal care, adoption or, if you want, for termination of the pregnancy.

❖ Sometimes sitting down quietly on your own and writing a list of all the reasons for or against each option is helpful.

❖ You'll have to be totally honest with yourself to do this and probably, it won't be easy.

❖ *Whatever* you decide you will have to live with your decision for life. You may need a lot of emotional support in the future.

❖ Don't be afraid to admit you feel scared. Let your tears come out and don't try to be brave about it all.

❖ Your decision will be right *for you* if you're strong enough to be honest with yourself. Although you may feel sad, look ahead and try to make something positive come out of what you may feel is a negative situation.

❖ If you decide to keep your baby, focus on being the best Mum in the world. You'll need lots of support and it'll be very hard work at times.

❖ If you decide to terminate or have the baby adopted, try to aim for something which you wouldn't have been able to do had you kept the baby; then *go for it* and do it really well.

❖ You may spend time going through a natural grieving process of anger, guilt, frustration, resentment and, finally, acceptance.

❖ Sometimes, it helps to talk your feelings through with someone; at other times, just writing down all your feelings, being very honest with yourself as you write, can be particularly helpful and healing, too.

❖ It takes some women a long time, others only a short time, to recover emotionally after terminating their pregnancy or giving their baby up for adoption. It depends on the circumstances surrounding your decision.

❖ Whatever course of action you decide upon, you will find that a lot of help is available, if you ask for it. Don't feel pressured into taking a particular decision.

Motherhood has its rewards but getting pregnant is the easy part. Having a baby is harder. Bringing up a child can be extremely difficult at times.

Protect yourself from pregnancy until you're REALLY sure you can support the consequences of your actions —in ALL ways.

There is no guarantee that your relationship will last or that you child will be healthy.

Be careful and BE SURE.

Sarah Moore
GeeStor Productions Ltd.

What about my partner?

❖ Your partner will also have emotions about it, if you've told him you're pregnant.

❖ Encourage him to talk, rather than bottle up his feelings.

❖ He may be confused, feel guilty and not know how to talk to you honestly, from fear of upsetting you.

❖ He may want you to terminate the pregnancy but not know how to tell you.

❖ He may want you to keep the baby – but, again, not know how to tell you.

❖ He may rant and rave and try to make you do the opposite of what *you* really want to do.

❖ He may, of course, be extremely supportive and, like you, may not know what he *really* wants you to do.

❖ He needs to be able to talk to someone, just as you do but, most men don't share their feelings as openly or easily as women.

❖ For him, too, the technique of writing all his feelings down, honestly and openly, may help.

❖ If he bottles up his feelings it could lead to emotional or physical problems eg. impotence and other sexual difficulties.

❖ Don't deny him his feelings. Even though he can't force you to do what you don't want with the pregnancy, it can be as emotionally traumatic for him as it is for you.

❖ This is a difficult decision but it must be yours and *yours alone*.

❖ For further support he could visit his Family Planning Clinic or GP for referral to a psychosexual therapist if there is not a *Well Man Clinic* in the area or nearby access to other counselling services.

I've heard that I won't be able to have a baby in the future if I have a termination. Is this true?

❖ A legal, surgical or medical termination *(abortion)* should not prevent you getting pregnant again.

❖ The greatest risk of infection/ infertility after termination is from an existing infection eg. *chlamydia* – which you are suffering from at the time of your operation. This could be pushed further into your body during surgery.

❖ Most reputable clinics now offer a test for *chlamydia* before surgery and some recommend that you go for an additional STI check up at a GUM clinic, to prevent post-operative complications.

There's no excuse left.

Condoms are free at Family Planning, Brook and GUM clinics.

They're open for men, too.

Check them out sometime and don't be silly with your Willy.

Eddie Nestor
Actor/Comedian

Men make sperm all the time, but can I run out of eggs if I have too much sex?

* No, you can't run out of eggs this way.
* You're born with your lifetime's supply of potential eggs in your ovaries.
* You gradually run out of them as you get older.
* Becoming pregnant can get more difficult as your age increases.
* Most women remain fertile until their menopause, which is usually around 50 years of age, when their periods stop.

I don't want to be like my Mum and have a baby when I'm a teenager, so what can I do?

* There's no need for you to repeat what happened to your mother.
* Wait until you're ready to bring a baby into the world.
* *For further information on contraception see pages 49-97*

Do women have erections?

* Yes, your clitoris becomes erect when you're sexually aroused.

I've heard that women make smegma. What is that?

* Smegma is a natural lubricant and, just as men make it in the tiny glands under their foreskin, you make it to keep the area around your clitoris comfortable.
* That's a good reason why it's important to wash your genital area and wear clean underwear every day.

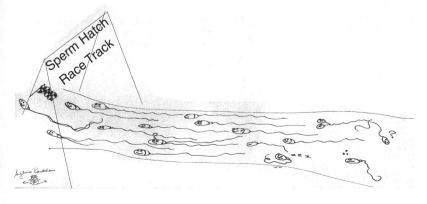

Should I get pain after sex?

- ❖ No, you shouldn't get pain after, or during, sex.
- ❖ If you get pain, which doesn't go if you change your sexual position, there could be a number of reasons.
- ❖ It's advisable to seek medical advice to make sure you don't have a pelvic infection eg. from *chlamydia* and/or *gonorrhoea*, in particular. They're infections (STIs) which can lead to *pelvic inflammatory disease* which can cause painful sex and lead to infertility – ie. being unable to get pregnant naturally.

If a pregnant woman has sex with someone who has VD will the baby be infected?

- ❖ VD (venereal disease) means sexually transmitted disease or infection. So yes, the baby is at risk of infection.

Pelvic infection

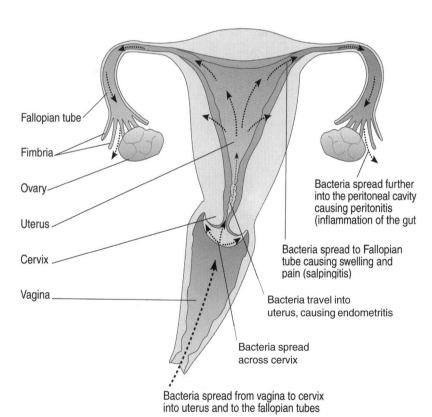

Fallopian tube

Fimbria

Ovary

Uterus

Cervix

Vagina

Bacteria spread further into the peritoneal cavity causing peritonitis (inflammation of the gut

Bacteria spread to Fallopian tube causing swelling and pain (salpingitis)

Bacteria travel into uterus, causing endometritis

Bacteria spread across cervix

Bacteria spread from vagina to cervix into uterus and to the fallopian tubes

SEXplained...® © 1999 Helen Knox

As a young woman, is it dangerous for my health if I have sex under the age of 16?

❖ You could become pregnant – which carries many risks.

❖ There's a high risk of infertility *(being unable to have a baby)* if you catch sexually transmitted infections, such as *gonorrhoea* or *chlamydia* and develop *pelvic inflammatory disease (PID)*.

❖ The neck of your womb *(cervix)* doesn't mature until you're about 23 years of age. Sometimes its delicate covering can be affected when not fully mature or developed – particularly if you catch certain varieties of the *genital wart virus* (HPV/human papilloma virus) from a partner or if you smoke. Both are thought to increase your risk of developing pre-cervical cancer.

Can I reduce these risks if I do have sex under the age of 16?

❖ If a condom or other barrier form of contraception – *eg. a diaphragm/ cap or Femidom® (female condom)* – is used properly each time, it can protect your cervix.

❖ It's better to wait until you're older and always use condoms.

Is it normal to bleed between my periods?

❖ No, bleeding on days when you wouldn't normally expect to bleed is not normal.

❖ If you're taking the Pill, check if you've forgotten any, had antibiotics, diarrhoea or vomiting, all of which can interfere with the effect of the Pill.

❖ If you've had sex with a new partner in the last three months, or you're not sure if your partner is faithful to you, seek medical advice. You may have caught an infection called *chlamydia*, have an abnormality at your cervix, or another medical condition which should be diagnosed properly.

I've heard that it can cause vaginal infections if I douche *(squirt fluid into my vagina to wash it out)* use bubble bath, vaginal deodorants, scented soaps, etc. Is this true?

❖ Yes, douching is not advisable. Your vagina is a self-cleansing area which doesn't need to be washed out.

❖ It's OK to use scented soaps or bubble-baths occasionally but don't overdo it.

❖ Vaginal deodorants aren't necessary and can cause irritation.

❖ Don't soak for too long in a very soapy bath because you could upset the normal acid conditions of your vagina and develop thrush or bacterial vaginosis.

❖ Just wash and dry yourself with mild soap and water externally *(outside)* rinse well, then towel dry.

❖ Wash daily or twice daily as preferred.

❖ Don't put talcum powder in your genital area either. It can get sweaty, sticky or smelly and isn't necessary.

I want my parents to know I'm sexually active and grown up enough to take precautions but I don't know how to tell them without them getting angry with me, as they probably won't approve.

❖ Just because you've had sex it doesn't necessarily mean you're grown up. Your parents love you and after they get over any initial shock, they'll realise you're being responsible seeking advice about contraception and/or infection.

❖ Some young people broach the subject by leaving contraception and safer sex leaflets lying around for their parents to find.

❖ That way, they can mention the subject to you instead and you can start talking about it together.

❖ Once any initial shock wears off, your parents might actually surprise you and be very supportive.

❖ You don't have to tell them about visiting your GP or FPC but some people suggest you do.

❖ Generally, your GP/Family Planning Clinic won't tell anyone without your permission, whatever your age.

❖ This service is confidential.

My parents get embarrassed when I ask about sex. Why, when they must have *done it* for me to be here?

❖ Not all parents feel comfortable talking about sex to children.

❖ Sometimes parents find it difficult to accept that you're growing up and developing your sexuality *(sexual preference)*.

❖ For many people talking about sex is still a taboo *(forbidden)* subject.

❖ Some adults simply don't know *how* to answer questions about sex properly. They avoid answering you to try and hide their embarrassment or ignorance!

Who else can I ask because I'm too embarrassed to ask my parents about sex?

❖ You can ask you Family Planning Clinic Doctor or Nurse, your School Nurse, GP or Practice Nurse, Teacher, Youth Worker, the FPA helpline or Childline.

❖ You may find it less embarrassing to talk to an aunt, uncle or another adult if you know they will answer you honestly.

❖ In the UK, apart from health authority Family Planning Clinics and specialist young people's services, the Brook Advisory Centres run contraception and advice sessions for young people.

❖ If the answer to your question isn't in this book – and you have access to the Internet – you can get confidential online Contraception and Sexual Health advice by visiting the **SEXplained...**® **Website** at **http://www.sexplained.com** or www.virgin.net/health *Ask the Experts.*

❖ Books and magazines are another popular source of information for many young people, too.

❖ *For further information see pages 182-183.*

Is it ok for me to have sex under the age of 16?

❖ In the UK and according to the *Sexual Offences Act 1956*, it's illegal for a male to have sex with a female who is a minor and is under the legal age to give consent *(permission)*. It would be classified as unlawful sexual intercourse *(USI)*.

❖ *For further information on Young People, Sex and the Law see page 121.*

Why don't parents mind boys having sex, but they mind girls having it? Surely this is unfair?

❖ It's unfair but it's universally accepted.

❖ Adults tend to be protective towards their daughters and feel that sons can look after their physical safety.

❖ A young man needs an erection to have sex, which he *can* learn to control.

❖ A young woman can get pregnant. She can also be forced, bullied or persuaded to have sex and is much more vulnerable.

❖ Unless a young woman has an abortion, or has the baby adopted, this often leaves Mum *holding the baby* while her daughter goes back to school to finish her education; or the young woman's life is put *on hold* until her baby goes to school etc.

❖ Most parents want their children to experience many things in life before becoming parents.

❖ Unfortunately, many young fathers are irresponsible and don't stay around for very long after their baby is born. They prefer their freedom!

Why do my parents still have sex?

❖ Presumably because they still love each other and enjoy the physical side of love and an active sex life together.

❖ It often goes hand in hand with having a happy relationship, so you should be pleased they still want to enjoy each other in this way.

❖ Having sex doesn't have to stop when you reach a 'certain age'.

❖ Believe it or not, you'll probably still want to have sex yourself when you are as old as they are!

If this is so, why do my parents mind my grandparents having sex?

❖ Just as you find it difficult to think of your parents still having sex, they may think the same way about *their* parents!

❖ Once they think it through, they'll realise there's nothing wrong with their parents making love and expressing their affection for each other in this way.

Kiss a safe practitioner and live to appreciate the difference.

Richard Ginn

I worry that I'm different from other young people. How can I tell, and who can I turn to for support?

❖ Generally, growing up is a very confusing time. It's complicated by sexual feelings and wonderings.

❖ Sexuality is not something anyone can tell by looking at you. Most people have wondered about their sexuality at some stage in their life – if they're honest.

❖ Some, live in great fear of what they don't want to admit to themselves; and others wonder only briefly about their sexual preference.

❖ Many young people experiment and play games of an overtly sexy nature. If, during sex play you experienced what you later consider to have been a homosexual encounter, that alone doesn't mean that you're gay, lesbian or bisexual.

❖ It's normal to be fond of a best friend of the same sex whilst you're growing up and you may want to spend all your free time with him or her.

❖ This may change as you grow more aware of the opposite sex and become attracted to its members.

❖ However, you may be one of the many people who don't become attracted to the opposite sex but remain attracted to members of your own sex/gender.

❖ Whatever the many theories about why this happens, it's important to accept that it's how you, yourself, feel.

❖ One of the most difficult things is learning to be honest with yourself and to overcome how you feel before telling anyone else.

❖ You may feel extremely confused, lonely, and even angry, that you're different from your friends who openly fancy members of the opposite sex and make a big show of it.

❖ You may be tempted to force yourself to have relationships with members of the opposite sex to hide your true feelings. You may greatly fear rejection by your peers or your family if you're open or 'come out' about your 'secret'.

❖ Some gay men or lesbians get married in the hope of forcing themselves into heterosexuality and perceived normality.

❖ They may then spend years in emotional turmoil before developing the courage to be honest with their partner about their sexual preference.

❖ Some people like to cross dress and wear the clothing usually associated with the opposite sex *(transvestite)*; while others want to change their sex and undergo years of medical treatment *(trans-sexual)*.

❖ Many are openly bisexual once they acknowledge their own feelings; others remain closet/secret bisexuals and seek pleasure outside their main relationship.

❖ This can be risky for both their health and their main relationship should their partner find out either by catching an infection or by some other means.

- ❖ When you're in a relationship, you have a responsibility towards your partner. It may be difficult but it's better to be honest than let your partner find out another way.
- ❖ These fears are very real and important to a young person experiencing the complicated adult world.
- ❖ The hardest person to lie to, in the end, is yourself.
- ❖ If you're still not sure about your sexuality, you may find a helpline in your area or a national helpline beneficial.
- ❖ Helplines offer a safe and anonymous way of discussing your fears with people who will listen and understand how you're feeling. They won't laugh at you or judge you.

- ❖ Alternatively, you may find your local library or bookshop a useful source of information.
- ❖ If you have access to the Internet you might find some of the 'chat programs' a useful and anonymous way of talking about your worries to other people of different ages.
- ❖ If a grown up of the same sex treats you in an obviously sexual way there are laws to protect you if you are under the legal age to give consent. *(In the UK, 16 for heterosexual sex and at present 18 for homosexual sex).*
- ❖ *For further information on Young People, Sex and the Law, see page 121-132.*

Don't believe all you hear – it's true what they say; girls that are easy to make laugh are even easier to get to lay down! – but guys, always wear a jacket.

Robbie Gee
Actor/Comedian

HM Prison

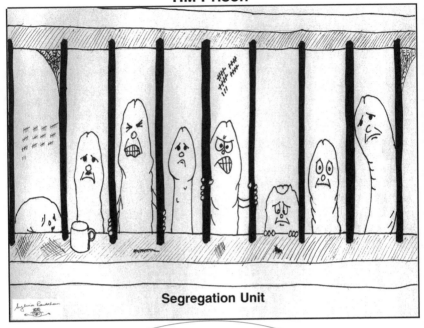

Segregation Unit

*I used to think I was invincible
and **respect** was something you earned.
I've hurt and upset too many people trying to get, so
called, respect. I even used to tool-up with a knife or gun to
make me appear something I wasn't. Having someone 'badder'
and bigger come ahead of me, now I see how the respect is taken from
me and given to him. What I thought was respect, was actually fear.
I was the one in fear – and I instilled fear in others for some cheap thrill.
I couldn't tell anyone how scared I really was, deep down inside.
Now look where I am. I'm wasting my life in prison when I should have been
living a good life and earning **genuine** respect. I regret a lot and just hope I can
start my life over again when I get out. This may be a University of Crime, but
crime is one subject I wish I'd dropped when I had the chance at school,
instead of rebelling all the time and thinking I was so smart
– and **they** were all fools. I've learned one heavy lesson here.
Don't dis other people 'cos you could end up here, too – and it ain't nice at all.
It's lonely. It's frightening. It's not the fun some so called 'rude boys' make it
out to be. They're liars. They're fools. I **have** to change my ways, 'cos I
don't **ever** wanna come back here. They all say that, I know – but
too many return. The arm of the Law really is long – and this
ain't no way to live.*
Anonymous in Prison
Dying of shame

According to the *Sexual Offences Act 1956*, it is an offence for a man to rape a woman or another man.

A man commits rape if:

(a) he has sexual intercourse with a person *(whether vaginal or anal)* who at the time of the intercourse does not consent to it: and

(b) at the time he knows that the person does not consent to the intercourse or is reckless as to whether that person consents to it.

Buggery/sodomy means

❖ Anal penetration with a penis.

Age of consent

❖ At present, in the UK, **the age of consent** for heterosexual vaginal sex is 16 and for homosexual *and* heterosexual anal sex is 18.

❖ In the UK, it's illegal for a male to have sex with a female who is a minor *(under the legal age to give consent/permission)*. It's classified as unlawful sexual intercourse *(USI)*.

❖ A child is someone under the age of 14.

❖ The age of consent and the Law varies in other countries and states.

❖ Currently, in the UK, lowering the age of homosexual consent is under review.

❖ *For further information on homosexual legal issues see Stonewall on page 182.*

The girl looked older

❖ In defence of having sex with a minor, some men state that the girl looked older but they may end up in trouble with the Law if she's under 16.

❖ Although the Law is clear, in practice, because of the *Children Act 1989* and the *Gillick Competency Ruling*, sex with young people can be a complicated area.

❖ If a male, over the age of 24 has sex with a female under 13, he faces a sentence of life in prison for unlawful sexual intercourse *(USI)*. The question of consent does not arise and without consent it is rape.

❖ If a male is over 24 and the female 14-16 it is rape *without* consent or USI *with* consent. He faces a maximum sentence of life in prison for rape or 2 years for USI.

❖ If a male is *under* the age of 24 and the female is between 14 and 16 years of age, it is unlawful sexual intercourse or rape. Age is sometimes used as an excuse unless he's been charged with a similar offence before.

Two teenagers having sex together

❖ If a 14 or 15 year old male and female have sex together, by mutual agreement, it's illegal but in practice is deemed *(considered)* a less serious offence. It's not wise though and something they may regret later. The young man is at risk of being charged with a sexual offence, for which he *could* be placed on the Sex Offenders Register and have to report to the Police.

Threats

❖ It is also an offence for a *person to procure (obtain) a female, by threats or intimidation, to have sexual intercourse.*

Drug rape

❖ It is an offence for *a person to apply or administer to, or cause to be taken by a female any drug, matter or thing with intent to stupefy (confuse) or overpower her so as thereby to enable any man to have unlawful sexual intercourse with her.*

❖ If a male has sex with a female who is asleep naturally or under the influence of alcohol or other drug(s) it is rape, for she is unconscious *(not awake)* and unable, therefore, to give consent.

❖ The maximum sentence for drug rape is life in prison.

Other people present

❖ Although she cannot commit rape, a female – or another male who is present at the time of a rape, commits an offence – and may be charged with aiding and abetting rape.

❖ It is legal for two people over the age of consent to have sex – but, if a 3rd party *(another person)* is present, it is a criminal offence, whether the group is heterosexual *or* homosexual.

❖ It is a criminal offence to have sex in a public place – or a private place if a 3rd party is present (heterosexual *OR* homosexual).

Lesbian offence

❖ Since a female under 16 cannot give consent, another female having lesbian sex with her commits indecent assault, which could carry a maximum sentence of 10 years in prison.

Property offence

❖ It is an offence for a property owner or occupier to allow his or her premises to be used for someone to have sex with a minor. If the female is under 13, he or she faces a maximum sentence of life in prison. If the female is under 16, he or she faces 2 years in prison.

At what age can I marry?

❖ In England, Wales and Northern Ireland a young person can marry from the age of 16 to 18 with parental consent and from 18 without parental consent.

❖ In Scotland, young people can marry from the age of 16 without parental consent.

Anal sex or buggery/sodomy

(a) Anal sex with a person – male or female – under the age of 16 or an older male or female without consent is illegal and carries a maximum sentence of life in prison.

(b) Anal sex, in the UK, between a consenting heterosexual OR homosexual couple is illegal between the age of 16 and 18 and carries a sentence of 2 years in prison.

(c) Anal sex under the age of 16, whether receiving or giving *with agreement*, the couple are both guilty in law and it carries a prison sentence.

Bestiality means:

* Bestiality means sex with an animal. It is illegal and carries a maximum sentence of life in prison.

Therefore:

* It's far safer to wait until you're older before having sex.
* It's better for a man to wait until there's no doubt whatsoever about a young woman's age before trying to have sex with her – with her agreement.
* Sometimes a young girl lies about her age when they fancy an older man. Being questioned by the Police about underage sex could be damaging to a man's reputation.
* There's no legal age of consent for heterosexual boys but it's illegal for a woman over 16 to have sex with or *interfere with* a young man under the age of 16.
* She can be prosecuted for indecent assault and faces a maximum sentence of 10 years in prison, the same as men.

What is abuse?

* Actual or threatened violence or abuse is usually by one person against another or others, as a quest for power over them and to make their victim do what they want.
* This may be by an adult against a child, a child against another child, adult to adult, child to adult or group/gang bullying.
* It can be male against male, male against female or female against male or female.

Abuse comes in many forms and is not just physical

* **Emotional abuse** – eg. constantly ridiculing *(poking fun at or belittling)* someone, instilling fear in or criticising them with or without the threat of using physical violence against them.
* **Physical abuse** – eg. hitting, punching, poking, slapping or pushing someone about.
* **Sexual abuse** – eg. rape; being forced to participate in humiliating sex acts; being shown or having access to pornographic material beyond your understanding; or being touched in a private place in a way which makes you feel uncomfortable.
* **Neglect** – eg. where you're left unattended, unfed and/or feel unloved.
* **Financial abuse** – eg. depriving someone of any money or refusing to pay bills, so that they're in fear of the gas or electricity being cut off or of going hungry.
* **Bullying** – eg. by other pupils at school is also abuse, as is having to watch domestic violence or be forced into any of these abuses, at home.

Always protect yourself.
Respect yourself.
Respect your partner.

Kat
Choreographer
& All Round Entertainer

Some of that has happened to me but I'm terrified to tell anyone. I'm scared they won't believe me and I'm scared I'll get into trouble if I tell. I can't stop having nightmares about what's happened. Where can I get help?

❖ As long as you don't ask the person abusing you, be brave enough to ask anyone else for help. **SPEAK OUT**.

❖ If the first person you turn to doesn't help you in the way you want, **KEEP ASKING UNTIL YOU GET THE HELP YOU NEED AND FEEL SAFE**.

❖ If the trouble is at home, tell someone outside the home, ie. your teacher – but if the trouble is from outside your home, tell your parents, trusted aunts, uncles or grandparents.

Other people to ask for help include:

❖ a neighbour you know well.

❖ a youth worker.

❖ the Police or social worker.

❖ Health visitor, GP, Practice Nurse or School Nurse.

❖ Childline or the Samaritans.

❖ NSPCC, Barnardos or Rape Crisis.

❖ your best friend, older cousin, brother, sister or someone else that you trust to help you.

❖ you may find that another member of your family is also a victim of abuse and equally scared to speak out, but with your help they may feel able to do so.

If a girl or woman says NO, does she really mean NO – or does she mean Yes?

❖ She means **NO** and don't think otherwise.

❖ If you say **No** do *you* mean Yes?

❖ By saying **NO** a girl or woman is stating that she does NOT give consent *(permission)* for whatever happens next.

❖ By taking no notice and carrying on, you're breaking the Law, acting recklessly and without due regard or care for your partner.

❖ If you don't stop you're committing a sexual offence.

But some girls say they mean YES when they say NO. It's very confusing

❖ As confusing as it may be, it's best and safest not to listen to them and simply *accept that NO means NO, and stop.*

❖ Even if you're about to ejaculate - **STOP**, otherwise you could get into serious legal trouble.

❖ It may not seem fair to have to stop – and it may even seem impossible but it could prevent you from ruining your life by going to prison and/or getting a criminal record with all the associated stigma attached to sex related crime. All for something you didn't mean to do!

❖ Sex by consent can be very enjoyable. Sex without consent is miserable and degrading.

❖ Stopping may make you feel confused, grumpy, annoyed, frustrated etc. but it could keep you safe and out of prison.

❖ This goes for all men, not just for young men embarking on a sexual journey.

SEXplained...® © 1999 Helen Knox

- You could be charged with rape if you misread the signals.
- No man is immune, however much you may think *It couldn't happen to me.*
- Take time to get to know some-one very well before you have sex together. Be clear about what your partner will or won't allow, before you start.
- If you change your mind during foreplay, state clearly that you don't want penetration. If you allow penetration, it's not rape for *that* individual incident.
- If, however, you/they get up, leave the room and return, it's a *separate* incident and you must not assume that you have permission to touch or have sex again, without consent. To do so, would be sexual assault or rape since it's a different incident from the first.

Recreational drugs, alcohol and taking advantage

- Young men, in particular, should be aware that it's a criminal offence to give alcohol or other drug to someone with the intention of having sex with them later.
- You risk being accused of rape or another sexual offence, should they later state that they didn't want to have sex with you.
- Whilst under the influence of alcohol or mind-altering drugs, inhibitions are likely to be reduced and casual, unprotected sex more than likely.
- This brings with it the serious risk of (a) pregnancy and (b) sexually transmitted infections.
- Remember; Emergency Contraception *is* available *(see pages 61-63).*
- The GUM/STI clinic can help diagnose/treat the infections you may worry about. However, it can't clear up some viral infections from your system.
- *For more information on date rape see pages 121 and 164.*

Ignorance doesn't pay for unplanned babies or the results of sexual diseases.
Lee Parker
Youth Worker, south London

Young People, Sex and the Law

I fancy my teacher *(youth worker or other adult I look up to)* and think I'm in love with him or her. Is this OK?

❖ Many young people get a crush on, or fancy, a teacher or another significant adult of either sex, whom they admire and can't imagine life without them around.

❖ In some ways it's a compliment you're paying that person.

❖ The teacher or other adult may realise you have a crush on them and should try to understand your feelings.

❖ They may be rather embarrassed when they realise how you feel but they should find a gentle way to discourage you from developing your feelings further, even if you'd like them to act differently towards you.

❖ They know more about the rights and wrongs of the world and until you're physically and emotionally mature and independent, they shouldn't do or say anything to let your crush lead any further – or take advantage of your feelings.

❖ They know they'd be breaking the Law if they developed the relationship in a physical way, if you're under 16 years of age.

❖ Most teachers are aware that this can happen and try their best not to hurt their pupils' feelings. At the same time, they keep a potentially troublesome situation from developing.

❖ As hard as it may sound, you have come into their life as part of their job, not as part of their family.

❖ They've been placed in a position of trust by your parents or guardians and have a responsibility towards you.

❖ They're not employed to love you, to lead your feelings on in any way, or make you feel that they could ever be more than a friend to you, in the adult role they hold.

❖ With time, these feelings fade and are diverted towards someone nearer your own age, with whom you can develop a more appropriate relationship.

❖ They may well remain as a cherished memory, reminding you of happier times at that particular school, and you will look back on their support as a best friend upon whom you could count for help and advice.

If an older guy wants to have sex with me but I'm under age and not ready, what should I do?

❖ Don't do it. It's illegal.

❖ Tell him you're under age and what he's suggesting is illegal.

❖ It's true and may make him realise the trouble he could get into with the Police.

❖ He could end up in prison on a rape charge, since you're under the legal age to give consent.

❖ In law, a male having sex with a female under the age of consent is committing unlawful sexual intercourse, and because you're under the age of consent, it's rape.

❖ It's no joke for a man to go to prison on a rape charge and it could be very dangerous for him.

❖ He'll be terrified of other prisoners finding out why he's there, since few people like child molesters – ie. someone who has sex with a minor.

❖ He should keep his penis in his pants and keep away from you until you're older and you can give your consent legally.

❖ Don't allow him to make you feel pressured.

❖ If he doesn't accept that, ask yourself whether you really want or need him in your life. It's obvious that what he really wants is sex; he doesn't care about you – just your body and his wants.

What if the person trying to have sex with me is a member of my own family?

❖ Sex with a member of your own family is called incest and it's against the Law *(illegal)*.

❖ If pregnancy occurs where there are blood ties between sexual partners it's genetically dangerous.

❖ Therefore, a man must not knowingly have sex with his mother, sister, daughter or grand-daughter. If the female is under 13 he faces life in prison. If the female is over 13 he faces 7 years in prison. There is NO question of consent in this case.

❖ A woman over 16 must not knowingly ALLOW her son, brother, father, grand- or great-grand father to have sex with her. To do so is illegal and could result in a prison sentence of 7 years. There is NO question of consent in this case.

❖ Although not incest, step-parents or other relatives have also been known to abuse young people. This is wrong so you must speak out about that, too.

❖ The Law is there to protect you, so get help from the Police, or a reliable adult, who will take it

further for you. Speak out to end the distress.

❖ By speaking out, when you feel ready and safe, you may be able to protect other family members from a similar kind of abuse.

❖ If the older person tells you to keep it a secret – or says that bad things will happen to you if you tell anyone – again, raise the alarm. This is a common way that the abuser terrifies in order to keep their victim under their control.

❖ Use the Law, get help and fight back, however scared you feel.

❖ If you're open and honest with the Police, you'll get lots of support. They won't force you to go to Court if you're too scared, even though your attacker should be locked away to prevent them hurting someone else. They have powers to make you go ahead, but your safety is their top priority. They're on YOUR side, so *do* talk to them.

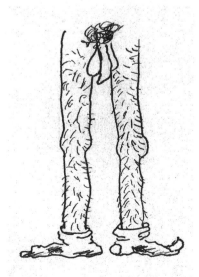

If I am going out with an older person should I tell my parents?

❖ Yes, you should tell your parents.

❖ You may not want to but it's better to tell them than let them find out some other way.

❖ If you feel they'll disapprove, try telling them gradually and let them get to know your friend.

❖ If they get to know him or her, they might not feel as uncomfortable about it as you expect or tell you not to continue the relationship.

❖ They're not really out to stop you having fun, just looking out for your safety, however hard this may be to accept.

❖ They probably realise that telling you not to do something is the best way to push you to do it and if they disapprove strongly, it would probably backfire on them and make you more determined to continue!

❖ Your parents know about many things that can happen when older people are involved that you're innocent about. How would you feel if *your* child hid the truth from you?

❖ If you can't tell them, ask yourself why, then ask yourself if you should really be doing whatever it is. The chances are that you shouldn't; so ask yourself why you're doing it and be honest with your answers.

She's a tease, look how she dresses, she's asking for it *(sex)*

❖ If she hasn't verbally requested sex, to assume any woman wants sex, just from the way she dresses, is ignorant and dangerous.

❖ It's absolute nonsense and commonly thrown as a defence by men who've failed to realise that there's a huge difference between *look – but don't touch* and the clearly spoken permission to touch.

❖ Whatever anyone chooses to wear is up to her/him.

❖ Although someone may dress in a provocative or sexy style, at no time does that give you the right to assume they're willing, or ready, to have sex with you.

❖ Nor does it give you the right to cross the boundary of good manners and decency towards them.

❖ A man is in complete control of his hands and his penis, what he does with them and where he puts them.

❖ Neither is it sufficient defense to cast aspurtions *(make bad comment)* on the way someone chooses to dress. To step from looking with admiration at someone to touching, assaulting or raping her/him because of how they're dressed is totally unacceptable. It's a criminal offence and punishable in Law.

I was abused when I was younger. Will I still be able to have a baby?

❖ Your chance of getting pregnant is unlikely to have been damaged.

❖ Don't assume you can't get pregnant. It's always wise to use a reliable method of contraception until you're ready to get pregnant.

❖ If, however, you were given a sexually transmitted infection – eg. *chlamydia* or *gonorrhoea* – which led to pelvic inflammatory disease *(PID)* you may need to see a gynaecologist for specialist advice.

❖ PID can lead to infertility but *there really is no difference between you and a girl who wasn't abused but caught these infections.*

❖ Not all adults are monsters, but of course, it's quite understand-able that your trust in those who should have been protecting you has been damaged.

❖ It's important not to bottle your feelings up or harm yourself – especially when you did nothing wrong. Try to find someone with whom you can share those painful feelings and start to rebuild your life in a positive way.

❖ If the abuser was a relative or family friend, it's very important to tell the Police what's happened, even if it's *off the record.* You can, of course, tell them when you are older and feel more able to cope.

❖ If you then decide *not* to press charges against your abuser the Police will, at least, know about a possible abuser.

❖ You can, however, press charges later.

❖ By speaking out, you may help them protect another victim.

❖ Most abusers are known to their victim and family.

❖ You may not be emotionally relaxed or feel comfortable talking about or having sex. If you'd like help from a specially trained psychosexual counsellor, your Family Planning Clinic or your GP can refer you.

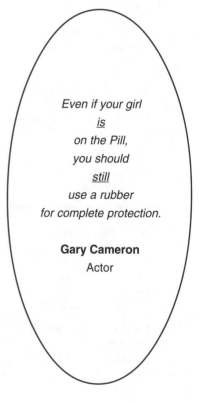

Even if your girl
is
on the Pill,
you should
still
use a rubber
for complete protection.

Gary Cameron
Actor

Since I was abused, I've hated myself. I don't trust other people or feel I'm worth loving but I desperately want someone to love me. Am I normal?

❖ Wanting to be loved is perfectly normal; everyone wants to be loved.

❖ For those who have been abused, it's natural to find it hard to trust other people.

❖ First, you have to learn to love yourself.

❖ You ARE worthy of love.

❖ When you start to believe this, you'll find that other people will respond to you in a more friendly way. Don't confuse sex with love. Sex and love can be totally separate requirements for *many* people.

❖ Be careful not to destroy yourself because of what someone did to you when you were younger.

❖ Learn to be in control of your feelings and fears. Don't let them rule you any longer.

❖ You CAN be happy again.

❖ Your GP or Family Planning Clinic can refer you to a specialist psychosexual counsellor who can give you time and help you work through your feelings.

If I have a baby, I'll have someone to love and someone who needs me, but they say I'm too young. Why do adults think like this?

❖ The adults probably say this because they've got the experience and are able to advise you from situations they've been in over the years.

❖ Your dream may seem wonderful but the reality is often less bright.

❖ Many young mothers wish they'd waited until they were older, although many do say they were glad they had their baby at that age.

❖ Having a baby is not a decision to make lightly. Your life will change forever.

❖ Not all men are reliable enough to provide for their partner and child.

❖ Your partner may walk away and leave you to cope alone. So don't assume he'll stay – you will need to plan accordingly.

❖ It's a fact of life that a man may promise to stick by you during pregnancy or when the baby's born. Promises may evaporate when your child becomes more demanding, when another woman comes along without the tie of a baby; and when he wants to have some fun without responsibility.

❖ If you don't have close family or friends with babies nearby, child care for times you want or need to go out alone can be very expensive.

❖ Don't rush into pregnancy; wait until you are sure of the support you'll receive.

❖ You should also consider the impact a baby will have on your education. Obtaining the necessary qualifications from school or college will put you in a better position to find employment. This will provide your baby with the security which he/she needs in addition to your love.

❖ It's very difficult to return to studying once you leave full-time education – particularly if you've been used to having some money in your pocket.

* Test your maternal instincts. Look after a friend's baby 24 hours a day, 7 days a week – then see how you feel.
* Alternatively, some educators have access to computerised teaching babies which behave, and display demands, just like those of a real baby. You may be able to borrow a teaching baby for a trial period so that you can see what it's like to have to respond to all its demands. But, unlike a real baby, you will be able to hand it back when you've had enough!
* A baby is a minimum 18 year commitment; expensive; hard physical and emotional work and not something to have for novelty value.
* When you're older, you will want a stable relationship. A partner might not be so attracted to someone who attracts the stigma of being a single parent on welfare.
* You cannot guarantee that your baby/child will be healthy all its life. This doesn't mean you'll love him/her any less but life can be extremely tough as a young parent under stress.
* Think very carefully before planning a baby. If you still decide to go ahead and have a baby, your life will change forever. Let's hope all your dreams come true.

What does a gardener do when planting seeds?

* A gardener plans ahead and takes time to nurture and prepare the area in which his seeds will grow.
* He waters and feeds the tiny plants and he works long and hard to ensure that they have the best chance of survival.
* After they grow, he still tends to their needs, protecting them from infection and harm.
* A baby deserves as much planning and forethought because you're planning the life of another human being, not just a plant.
* If, after careful planning and a lot of saving you still think this is what you want to do, then seek medical advice about pre-conceptual *(pre-pregnancy)* care.
* You'll need to be healthy during the first three months of your pregnancy, have vaccinations to protect your baby from miscarriage, blindness or deafness etc. – in case you come into contact with some-one who has rubella *(German measles)*.
* You'll need pre-natal care throughout your pregnancy to check that the baby is growing well and is healthy. This is particularly important if you have a medical condition that could be made worse by pregnancy. You'll also be advised to take folic acid tablets regularly before and during pregnancy.

I want someone to love me so I have sex and lots of one-night stands with lots of people. Is this OK?

- ❖ Simply having sex with someone doesn't mean they love you.
- ❖ After a while, you'll probably feel *used* or *abused* if you continue to search for love in this way.
- ❖ You may get a temporary ego boost when you feel that someone finds you attractive enough to have sex – but not much more.
- ❖ Except that, the more people you have sex with, the greater your risk of catching a sexually transmitted infection.
- ❖ Take time to get to know some-one very well before you have sex. It's safer and, in many ways, more healthy for you physically and emotionally than just having sex because you crave affection. Don't confuse the act of sex, with the act of love.

Penis manners maketh the man – and pleaseth the partner.

Penny Hopkinson
Editor & friend

All my friends go to parties and have sex with other people. I don't want to have sex, but my friends put pressure on me. I feel left out because I haven't done it yet. What should I do?

- ❖ Check out any venue where you don't know the host/ess. If you feel uncomfortable, don't go in.
- ❖ It is illegal for people to have sex
- (a) in a public place.
- (b) if a third party is present.
- ❖ If you feel uncomfortable, don't go in.
- ❖ If you find yourself in a club – or at a party where people are having sex – don't feel you have to have sex just because your friends do – or because you are there.
- ❖ Having sex is neither compulsory nor a kind of competition.
- ❖ Don't allow anyone to pressurise you into having sex.
- ❖ Secretly, your friends might be jealous that you still have your virginity and want to save it for later.
- ❖ Studies show that the majority of young people who have sex wish they'd waited until they were older before they started.
- ❖ Listen to your heart, not the bullies!

- ❖ **Male circumcision** is almost always carried out during the first two months of life when a baby boy is too young to remember what's happened.
- ❖ The foreskin *(prepuce)* or loose skin which covers the glans penis, is surgically removed; perhaps under local anaesthetic.
- ❖ It is widely practised in Jewish and Moslem communities for religious reasons; and it may be medically indicated later in life if the foreskin becomes inflamed and difficult to retract *(pull back)*. This is called *phimosis* and is often caused by poor genital hygiene.

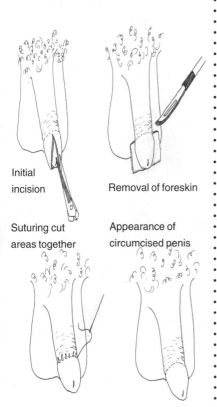

Initial incision

Removal of foreskin

Suturing cut areas together

Appearance of circumcised penis

- ❖ **Female circumcision** is still carried out, today, in some Moslem countries in Africa. It is also practised in other areas, but to a lesser extent. It is a traditional but barbaric *(brutal)* practise, for which there is no medical need whatsoever.
- ❖ It's also called female genital mutilation *(FGM)* due to the severe and totally unnecessary damage that's done to a young woman's genitalia. It is usually carried out between 7 and 11 years of age. The girls live the terror and pain of the procedure without anaesthetic, for life.
- ❖ In 1996 the World Health Organisation defined FGM as *any procedure which involves partial or total removal of or injury to the external genitalia, whether for cultural or other non-therapeutic (medical) reasons*.
- ❖ It will take years and a lot of education to ensure this practice is outlawed.
- ❖ It can involve removal of the prepuce *(skin covering the clitoris)* or removal of the clitoris itself *(clitaroidectomy)*.
- ❖ Quite often the labia minora *(vaginal lips)* are cut off.
- ❖ Sometimes the damage is so severe that almost all of the young woman's external genital area is removed and the raw areas sewn together, allowing only a small hole for urine and menstrual blood to pass through. *(This is called infibulation.)*

Left:

diagram of one technique of male circumcision – removal of foreskin (prepuce)

- ❖ It's carried out to ensure that the female will never enjoy sex and in the belief that her lack of enjoyment will prevent her from being unfaithful. The theory is that because she won't get *turned on* sexually, she won't look for boys and will remain faithful. However, since a woman finds sex painful and without pleasure she may inevitably look elsewhere, thinking that their husband is a useless lover!
- ❖ Girls often bleed to death from this mutilation – or from the septicaemia *(blood poisoning)* caused by dirty instruments or the techniques used to perform the circumcision.

- ❖ Sex can hurt these young women, and childbirth can be excruciatingly painful with the added risk of tearing, bleeding and infection.
- ❖ Traditionally, older women perform it on young girls before they reach puberty.
- ❖ In the West, it's viewed as cruel and as a form of child sex abuse as well as GBH *(grievous bodily harm)*.
- ❖ In London and other major cities, there are some specialist clinics where women can have surgery to undo as much of the damage as possible.
- ❖ Gradually the labia start to regrow – but not the clitoris.
- ❖ Lack of sexual enjoyment and the psychological scarring related to female circumcision, also remain for life.

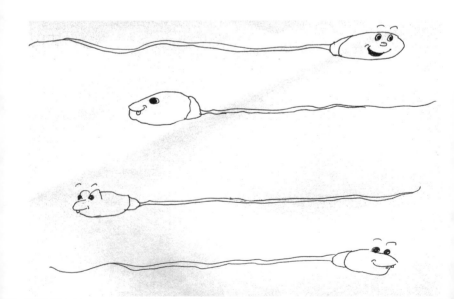

Many people have infections without realising – therefore the aim of this section is to ensure you are protected from all sexually transmitted infections not just HIV/AIDS.

Here are some facts

❖ In the tiny amount of blood involved in a needle stick injury *(stab or scratch with a syringe)* the chance of getting HIV, if it's present, is less than 1 in 300 *(0.3%)*.

❖ BUT — if they're present, the chance of getting Hepatitis B is 1 in 3 *(30%)* and/or Hepatitis C is 1 in 10 *(10%)*.

❖ HIV dies quickly in the open air compared with Hepatitis B which can live for up to 2 weeks in dried blood and Hepatitis C for up to 3 weeks.

❖ HIV has been found to live for 4 weeks or more in an infected syringe.

Think about this!

❖ Doctors, Nurses, Dentists and Surgeons take universal precautions – ie. they wear latex gloves, masks etc. – to protect themselves. They treat all patients the same – ie. as if there's a risk of infection.

❖ It's sensible to assume that the same unknown risk is present when you have sex. So protect yourself, since they each involve contact with the blood or body fluids of another person.

❖ Certain sexual activities take place which aren't usually discussed openly by young people. The following is an assessment of the level of risk involved according to the sexual activity.

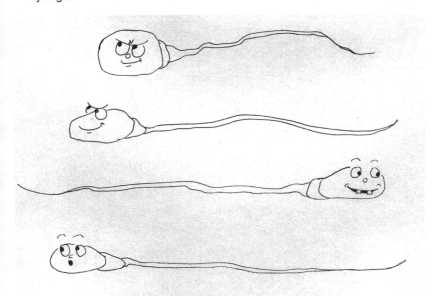

Safer Sex SEXplained...®

Highest risk activities include

❖ Anal sex *(buggery/sodomy)* without a condom.
❖ Vaginal sex without a condom.
❖ Giving oral sex *(a blow job/ fellatio)* to a man if his ejaculate enters your mouth.
❖ Giving oral sex to *(going down on/cunnilingus)* a woman during her period.
❖ Finger insertion *(anal or vaginal)* if there are cuts, sores, bleeding piles *(haemorrhoids)* or your partner has a period.
❖ Withdrawal *(pulling out)* before ejaculation, without wearing a condom.

Medium/high-risk activities include

❖ **Med/high**: Giving unprotected oral sex to a man without taking his ejaculate into your mouth.
❖ **Med/high**: Giving unprotected oral sex to a woman without her period.
❖ **Med**: Vaginal or anal sex with a condom.
❖ **Med**: Finger insertion *(anal or vaginal)* is safer if broken skin, cuts, sores etc. are covered with waterproof plaster.
❖ **Med**: Giving oral sex to a man who's wearing a condom.
❖ **Med**: Performing oral sex during a period but using a barrier as protection between your mouth and her body fluids. You can use a dental dam or cut a flavoured condom lengthwise and open it out as a barrier. Some people use microwave cling film, even though some germs can penetrate *(get through)* the plastic of cling film. *For further information on Dental Dams see page 139.*

❖ **Med**: Wet kissing *(deep French kissing)*. Safety depends upon the health of your lips and mouth and those of your partner*(s)*. If there are bleeding gums from newly brushed teeth or gum irritation caused by cut lips, cold sores *(herpes simplex)*, mouth ulcers or even from smoking cocaine, hepatitis can be passed this way – if it's present in blood stained saliva.

Low risk activities and alternatives to penetrative sex include

❖ Masturbating on your own.
❖ Masturbating your partner *(heavy petting)* but, if any part of your hand enters their body you should make sure that cuts, rashes or sores are covered by waterproof plaster or latex gloves beforehand.
❖ Dry kissing.
❖ Hugging.
❖ Love bites.
❖ Sexual arousal; fully clothed and remaining so!
❖ Anything else you can think of which doesn't involve the exchange of body fluids and gives mutual *(both of you)* pleasure by consent *(with permission)*.

Even though it's unrealistic, the safest kind of sex is no sex at all! Safer sex is the same for everyone, whether you're:

* **Straight** – a man who's sexually attracted to women or a woman who is sexually attracted to men *(heterosexual)*.
* **A gay man** – a man who's sexually attracted to other men *(homosexual)*.
* **Lesbian** – a woman who's sexually attracted to other women.
* **Bisexual** – someone who is sexually attracted to both men and woman.
* **Transvestite** – someone who habitually likes to wear clothing associated with the opposite sex.
* **Trans-sexual** – someone who firmly believes that they belong to the opposite sex, and may undergo *gender reassignment surgery* after thorough medical assessment, to make their external genitalia conform to their view of themselves.

Is oral sex when you *talk dirty* to each other?

* It could be but it also means mouth to genital contact.
* Oral sex to a man is called fellatio.
* It's commonly called a *blow job* – but you don't blow – you lick then suck his penis.
* Oral sex to a woman is called *cunnilingus* and you lick or gently suck her genital area – primarily her clitoris.
* It can give your partner enough sexual pleasure so that they reach orgasm. Some people prefer to perform oral sex rather than have penetrative sex. Other people don't enjoy it and prefer not to do it at all.

At the end of the day, buy a condom.
No sex is worth dying for.

Richard Blackwood
Comedian/MTV Presenter

Safer Sex SEXplained...®

Is it OK not to want oral sex?

❖ Yes, it's quite OK not to want oral sex.

❖ If you don't fancy it, simply tell your partner you'd prefer not to do it.

❖ Tell them gently so that they don't feel you don't want *them* (*rejected*). It's simply that you don't want to *do* something they might like to do with you.

❖ Never allow anyone to pressure you into oral sex. If you're going to do it there are some things you may not realise.

(a) In the context of a long-term, loving, trusting and totally monogamous *(one partner only)* relationship, where each of you has been fully tested for any STIs before you have sex together, oral sex is a fairly safe, low risk type of sex.

(b) Sore throat germs can still pass either way although the risk of catching *NSU, thrush* or *bacterial vaginosis* is minimal.

(c) The risk of infection increases considerably, if you have casual sex with someone you later find out has *gonorrhoea, chlamydia, herpes, warts, hepatitis, syphilis* – or any other sexually transmittable infection – in their mouth.

(d) If you're unfaithful to your partner, you risk being found out if you transfer an infection to them after having unprotected oral sex with someone else. That is in spite of using a condom for genital/penetrative sex!

(e) Since each STI can be caught in, or transferred from, someone's mouth to your genitalia – or from their genitalia to your mouth –

flavoured condoms are recommended when giving oral sex to a man *(a blow job/fellatio)*. Dental dams are advised when giving oral sex to *(cunnilingus/go down on)* a woman or if you lick your partner's anus *(anilingus/rimming)*.

(f) Alternatively, you can cut a flavoured condom along one side, open it out and place this over their genital area before oral sex, if you don't have a dental dam.

(g) Hepatitis B and Hepatitis C viruses can be present in infected blood and blood-stained body fluid and are much easier to catch than HIV.

❖ If you don't know whether your partner has hepatitis or not, you should ensure that cuts and sores on your fingers are be covered with waterproof plaster or latex gloves *before* you start any genital foreplay.

❖ It's considered good sexual manners to wash your genital area before you receive oral sex.

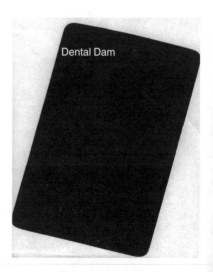

Dental Dam

Can I use flavoured condoms for penetrative sex?

❖ Yes you can have penetrative sex with a flavoured condom quite safely.

❖ **BUT – if you wear lipstick** when performing oral sex, change the condom before having penetrative sex, since lipstick rots latex.

❖ **If you don't wear lipstick**, you're safe to go from giving oral sex to having penetrative sex with the same condom.

❖ You may need to use extra lubricant to make sex more comfortable if the flavoured lubrication has come off – since a dry condom can cause stinging and general discomfort.

❖ *For further information on lubricants, see page 154-155.*

Does oral sex make a young woman pregnant?

❖ No, it doesn't make a woman pregnant.

What is the 69 position?

❖ The 69 position is one of the common positions used by a couple when having oral sex.

❖ You may face each other's feet and curl round to enable you to reach each other's genital area with your mouth.

❖ You then look like a 6 and 9 in position – hence the 69 position.

❖ It's also known as the Ying and Yang position and soixante-neuf.

See left:
Dental Dam

What are dental dams, I've never heard of them, neither have my friends?

❖ Just as you would use condoms routinely when having penetrative sex, it's sensible to protect your mouth when giving oral sex to your partner; or from being passed an infection they may have in their mouth.

❖ Flavoured condoms should be worn over a penis when giving oral sex to a man *(blow job/ fellatio)*.

❖ Originally, dental dams were simply sheets of latex *(rubber)* used by Dentists, until someone decided to use them as barrier protection to keep their mouth safe during oral sex.

❖ They're squares or oblongs of latex *(rubber)* which are placed over the whole genital area of a woman, or the anal area of a man, before they receive oral sexual stimulation.

❖ They're expensive, should be used only once and don't have a *use this way up* sign on them. So you might want to mark them, yourself. Otherwise, if the dam falls off and you replace it without checking, you could put it back the wrong way round, which would defeat the object of using it in the first place!

❖ Alternatively, make your own by cutting a flavoured condom from base to tip, then open it out to make a latex barrier. In an emergency, you could use some microwave cling film but this doesn't give as much protection as latex.

❖ See also *jel charging* on page 148.

What if the woman tells me not to use condoms because she doesn't like them?

- ❖ It's simple; don't enter her!
- ❖ If she won't use condoms with you, it's more than likely she hasn't used them with her previous partner(s)!
- ❖ Do you really want to receive all their germs?
- ❖ Tell her: *Sorry, no condoms, no sex. Try elsewhere. I value my Dick!*

What if a man tells me he doesn't and won't wear a condom?

- ❖ It's simple; don't let him enter!
- ❖ If he won't use condoms with you, it's more than likely he hasn't used them with his previous partner(s)!
- ❖ Do you really want to receive all their germs?
- ❖ Tell him: *Sorry, no condoms, no sex. Try elsewhere. I value my tubes!*

If I carry condoms, does this mean I'm promiscuous (*easy/slack/sleep around*)?

- ❖ No, it doesn't. If you're sexually active, it means you're mature enough to take responsibility for your health and safety – if of course, that you use them!
- ❖ Your partner may not be sufficiently organised to protect you both.
- ❖ If you're not sexually active at least you have the right idea about protecting yourself when you do have sex.
- ❖ Respecting yourself and your partner's health is an important step to maturity.
- ❖ Some grown-ups dislike touching a condom. But being familiar with the feel of condoms, to show off to your friends – even if it shocks your parents – is an important step in learning to look after yourself. It's good safer sexual practice.

Respect yourself.
Respect your partner.
It ain't good
to be an unplanned babyfather.

Gary Cameron
Actor

Should I practise using a condom on my own?

❖ Yes, everyone should know how to use a condom.

❖ Practise using a condom until you can wear it quickly and correctly. Most young men wake up with an early morning erection due to their last sexy dream of the night. Take advantage of this and practise, practise, practise!

❖ If you're skilled at putting one on:

(a) you'll be less embarrassed with a new partner;

(b) you'll be less likely to make a mistake; or for the condom to fail. It became a forgotten art when the Pill became widely available.

❖ Most men *(even adults)* don't know how to use a condom properly. This may sound odd, but many men weren't brought up to assume responsibility for pregnancy prevention.

❖ You're a long way ahead of the competition if you know how to use a condom correctly – and, who knows, by preventing infection/practising safer sex, you could also protect your life!

Should young women learn how to use condoms?

❖ Yes. Both men and women should be skilled at rolling on responsibility.

❖ Too few boys and men know how to use condoms correctly – so, it's vital that all women learn why and how they should be used.

❖ Many women learn the skill by practising on a large carrot, courgette or similarly shaped object!

When should male condoms be used?

❖ Male condoms should be used to prevent pregnancy/infection.

❖ It's vital that a condom is used before there is *any* genital contact whatsoever with your partner.

❖ There are approximately 3,000,000 sperm in the clear fluid which forms at the tip of an erect penis.

❖ That's enough to cause pregnancy and/or pass germs in the right conditions, without even penetrating *(entering)* your partner.

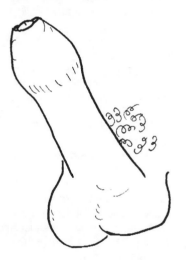

Important tips before you use a condom:

How are male condoms used?

(a) Wash any massage oils, baby oil or creams off your penis, using soap and water. Oils and latex/rubber do not mix and will break/rot/burst or split the condom and you will not be protected against pregnancy or infection.

(b) Check the expiry date on the packet and make sure that the condom meets recognised standards – ie. see if the box is marked with the British Standards kite mark, European *(CE)* mark, EN600 or the international standard of the country of origin.

(c) Before taking a sealed condom from the packet, check that the wrapping hasn't been damaged.

(d) Gently tear the wrapping to expose the condom. *Don't use your teeth!*

(e) Look at or feel the condom, to check which way round its going to unroll.

(f) Check that the teat *(reservoir)* is easy to hold or if it doesn't have a teat, make your own by squeezing the top 2.5 cms *(1 inch)* of the condom, to empty the air.

(g) Take the condom from its wrapping and hold the teat as you place it on the top of your own or your partner's fully erect penis.

(h) Unroll it, outwards and down over your/his penis for at least 5 cms *(2 inches)* before letting go of the teat. This will ensure that no air slips back into the teat. If it does, the condom may burst.

(i) Continue unrolling it over your penis until you reach your pubic hairline.

(j) Check that you have more than one condom – in case one fails or you make a mistake.

During sex

❖ It's sensible to check that the condom hasn't slipped slightly, as if it's coming off your penis. You will notice this from a slight change in sensation.

❖ If the condom has slipped, simply guide it back onto the shaft of your penis and continue.

❖ Re-lubricate, as necessary, using only water based lubricant.

❖ If you have sex for a long time – say more than ten minutes, or less if your partner isn't sufficiently moist/turned on – the condom may become too dry and will weaken. Also, your partner may become sore from dry friction and movement. To overcome this problem, you will need to use extra water based lubricant.

❖ *For further information about lubricants see page 154-155.*

After ejaculation

❖ You must ensure that the condom is held on your penis during withdrawal and that you withdraw *before* your penis starts to go soft/limp.

❖ If you don't, there's a greater chance that the condom may slip off and sperm may spill inside your partner.

❖ This would mean that using the condom was a waste of time and you would risk pregnancy/infection.

* Condoms should be used once only.
* After use, the condom should be wrapped it in a tissue and thrown in the bin. Condoms float, so don't try to flush them down the toilet.

If anything goes wrong

* If the condom splits or comes off before withdrawal, remember emergency contraception. The STI/GUM Clinic can help if you are worried about infection.
* *For further information on Emergency Contraception see page 61-63*

What if it won't roll right down?

* Check that the condom is round the right way – and not inside out. If it's inside out, throw it away and start again with another.
* Longer condoms are available from specialist suppliers. These may be more suitable.
* *For further information on condom suppliers see page 183.*

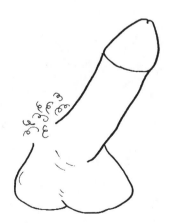

What if I make a mistake and put it on inside out?

* If this happens, throw it away *immediately*.
* Do not turn it over and try again because any sperm or germs are transferred directly inside your partner, risking pregnancy and/or infection.
* If that was your last condom, don't take the risk of having unprotected sex. Stop and consider the consequences.
* Carry at least one spare condom!

It bursts, it leaks and it doesn't feel the same, why?

* If your partner is not sufficiently moist or lubricated, the condom will dry out. This will make it sore to use and more likely to burst from increased tension and friction.

What if I don't get all the air out of the teat?

* Air in the teat is said to be a contributing factor when condoms fail.
* The pressure of ejaculation against the trapped air is thought to weaken the rubber and make the condom more likely to burst – usually along the shaft of the penis.

What if I have long nails, hang nails or rough nails?

* Be careful, your nails could puncture the rubber.

Condoms are too small for me, so I can't wear them

❖ A few years ago you might have got away with the excuse that condoms are too small! Today, there's a huge range from which to choose.

❖ Try various brands, until you find one that suits you.

❖ Changing to a thinner condom on which the ring is not so tight might make it more comfortable to wear.

❖ Condoms come with short teats, long teats or no teats; straight sides, flared sides; baggy tips or tight fit; with or without spermicide; with or without lubricant; various colours and flavours; various thickness; with or without ribbing; and different lengths. There are also hypo-allergenic condoms; polyurethane condoms; and condoms made from natural lamb membrane, so try each until you find one that suits you.

❖ With the introduction of the new European Standard *(CE)* condoms are 10mm *(½ inch)* longer and range in width from 88mm to 128mm in circumference.

Condoms are too big for me, what should I do?

❖ Smaller or tighter condoms are available.

❖ If you're young and they're too big for you, you could wait until you've fully grown before you have sex and are physically mature.

❖ Condoms are available to accommodate all sizes of mature penis.

❖ *Further information is available at a Family Planning Clinic, a pharmacy or from a specialist mail order condom supplier – see page 183.*

Some men suggest

❖ Try thicker condoms, if you are concerned about ejaculating too quickly *(premature ejaculation)*.

❖ Try tighter/smaller condoms or jel charging the condom if you are concerned about a delay in ejaculation. This may help you ejaculate more easily.

❖ *For further information on jel charging see page 148.*

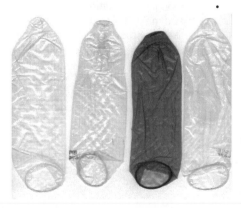

Condoms in various sizes - from small to extra large.

There are quality condoms to fit all size penises!

I'm allergic to condoms

❖ Hypo-allergenic *(low allergy)* condoms are available.
❖ It may not be the condom but the lubricant on it that's causing your discomfort.
❖ Try changing from condoms with spermicide on them *(nonoxynol 9 or 11)* to condoms which are lubricated only.
❖ Dryness can make sex very uncomfortable for both partners with or without condoms.
❖ To reduce discomfort, use a lot of extra water-based lubricant in case the allergy is friction based – ie. from being too dry.
❖ *For further information see 'Are there any new male condoms?' on page 146.*

What's spermicide?

❖ Spermicide is a chemical which kills sperm.

Spermicidal pessaries
Solidified spermicide which melts at body temperature.

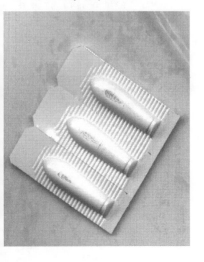

Should I use extra spermicide with condoms?

❖ Some studies show that by using extra spermicide you can reduce the risk of catching sexually transmitted infections. But with frequent use this may cause irritation in some people, particularly sex workers *(prostitutes)*.
❖ You'd also have slightly more protection against unplanned pregnancy if your condom split or came off.
❖ Some people however, are allergic to spermicide, in which case it might be wise to use a thicker, non-spermicidally lubricated condom.
❖ *For further information of Emergency Contraception see pages 61-63.*

Should I use spermicidally lubricated condoms or non-spermicidally lubricated ones?

❖ It doesn't matter which type you use. Spermicide can sometimes cause irritation. Some people think they're allergic to condoms when they are just reacting to the spermicide.
❖ Using a non-spermicidally lubricated or flavoured condom for vaginal penetrative sex correctly is thought to be equally effective. It may also be more comfortable for some people.
❖ It's important to use extra lubricant with either type of condom when it becomes dry and uncomfortable. This reduces any discomfort.

Should I use extra lubricant with condoms?

❖ Using extra lubricant is very wise indeed, since a dry or poorly lubricated condom can cause problems.

❖ It's especially important if you are having sex for a long time and the condom begins to dry out.

❖ A dry condom can be uncomfortable for both partners. It is more likely to burst, can cause tiny friction burns and may cause thrush to develop.

❖ Use only water-based lubricants, spermicidal creams or jel from a reliable sales outlet or Family Planning Clinic. NEVER use oil-based products with latex *(rubber)* condoms. They can ONLY be used with the polyurethane female condom *Femidom® (Reality®)* or the male condom, *Avanti®.* Neither product contains latex so cannot be damaged by oil.

If I wear two condoms, I'll be double safe, won't I?

❖ No, you won't be twice as safe.

❖ Although this is suggested in some parts of the world, condom manufacturers certainly don't recommend wearing two condoms at a time.

❖ In fact, condoms may be more likely to fail if used this way.

❖ Use the extra or ultra strong variety of condom instead.

Which condom can I use for anal sex?

❖ In many parts of the world anal sex is illegal.

❖ Anal sex became legal in the UK between consenting hetero-sexual couples over the age of 18, in April 1995. Currently it is legal between consenting homosexual couples over the age of 18. (This is under review at present.)

❖ No condom is licensed for anal sex, because no anal sex standards exist.

❖ Extra strong/ultra strong varieties of condom, which are slightly thicker, used with extra *water based lubricant* are recommended. These condoms are not spermicidally lubricated, because this may cause irritation.

❖ *For further information of homosexual legal issues see Stonewall on page 182.*

Are there any new male condoms?

❖ Yes, there's a polyurethane condom available, called Avanti®.

❖ It's more expensive than latex/rubber condoms.

❖ The main differences and/or advantages are:

(a) any lubricant can be used with it – not just water-based ones.

(b) it doesn't stretch as much as a latex condom.

(c) it is much wider.

(d) greater sensitivity can be expected.

(e) the polyurethane hardly smells.

(f) it's ideal for men or women who are allergic to all forms of latex, including the hypo-allergenic *(low allergy)* condoms.

❖ You must be careful to hold it on your penis after each ejaculation, when withdrawing after penetrative sex.

Ladies, please note!

❖ If you wear nail polish when you put a spermicidally lubricated condom onto your partner, use spermicide with your cap, or diaphragm, the spermicide may soften your nail polish.

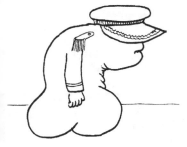

To all men and women

❖ NEVER use an oil-based lubricant with rubber/latex condoms. Oil based lubricants can damage the latex.

❖ Use water based lubricants ONLY or they will perish *(rot)* the latex in a very short time and make the condom more likely to burst.

❖ A damaged condom could put you at risk of pregnancy and/or infection.

❖ Water based lubricants are safe and can be washed off your hands with only water.

❖ Vaseline, baby oil, massage oil, lipstick, petroleum jelly, hand cream, suntan oil, butter, margarine, or anything which needs soap and water to wash off your hands MUST NOT BE USED with latex condoms.

❖ If any oil gets onto your penis before sex *(massage oil etc.)*, it must be washed off with soap and water before the condom is put on. This is because there may be enough oil left on the penis to rot the condom!

❖ If you think you are at risk of sexually transmitted infections you should visit a GUM/STI clinic – and particularly if you if you notice any unusual lumps, bumps, discharges, smells or sores in your mouth or genital area after sex.

❖ Seek help if you're worried in *any* way.

❖ Remember: Emergency Contraception is available should the condom fail.

❖ *For further information on Emergency Contraception see page 61-63.*

What's jel charging?

❖ Jel charging is when you put a small amount of water-based lubricant inside the tip of a condom before putting it on.

❖ Remember to expel the air carefully from the top 2.5 cms *(1 inch)* as the condom is rolled over your penis.

❖ Massage the lubricant over the glans *(helmet/hood)* of your penis.

❖ Be careful not to get lubricant down the shaft of your penis as moisture is more likely to make the condom slip off.

❖ The extra moistness of jel charging is said to greatly increase sensation, especially for circumcised man.

❖ If you're uncircumcised, hold your foreskin right back before putting on a condom. You may not require additional lubricant to enhance the sensation.

❖ Some men say that jel charging is *wetter and better than sex without a condom*.

❖ Your partner should add extra lubricant regularly to prevent the condom drying out during sex – and breaking when thrusting for a long time.

❖ Jel charging may seem a bit of a nuisance but, if it's built in to foreplay, it can add enjoyment by increasing the sensation!

❖ Make sure you become skilled at jel charging *before* you need to use a condom.

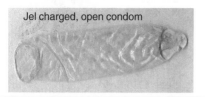

Jel charged, open condom

What is Femidom® the female condom?

❖ Known as Reality® in some countries, it's a relatively new type of contraceptive.

❖ It looks like a cross between a contraceptive cap and a loose condom.

❖ It should be used once only.

❖ It's made of pre-lubricated polyurethane.

❖ It's inserted into the vagina, although part of it stays outside to cover the external genital area. It covers the clitoris, so oral sex is safer. There's no need to use a dental dam.

❖ *Any* lubricant can be used with it.

❖ Your partner can keep his penis inside you after ejaculation, and when his penis goes soft.

❖ They're more expensive than male condoms – but are sometimes provided FREE at Family Planning Clinics.

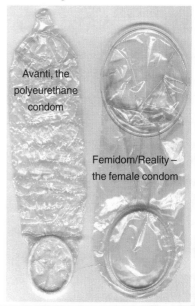

Avanti, the polyeurethane condom

Femidom/Reality – the female condom

Safer Sex SEXplained...®

How do I negotiate having safer sex when we *haven't* been using condoms but have been together a long time?

❖ This can be tricky!
❖ You could simply tell your partner that this is what you want to do, from now on. But how will they react?
❖ It's a question you will have to discuss together and examine your reasons for asking, very honestly.
❖ Introducing this question into your relationship for other reasons can be extremely difficult and is loaded with emotion.

You may have been advised or wish:

(a) to change from other methods of contraception to condoms for medical reasons.
(b) to use protection in addition to the Pill.
(c) to take a rest from the responsibility of birth control and want to pass this to your partner.
(d) because it's now routine practise for Family Planning staff to recommend a *Double Dutch* approach – ie. use condoms plus another method of birth control – plus the routine use of extra spermicide.
(e) your partner and furnishings stay drier after sex, as the ejaculate is contained within the condom!

Opposite – left to right:
comparison of male and female condom
Far left –
jel charged, open condom

What might this question imply if your partner asks you to use a condom?

❖ Would it mean
– *I don't trust you to be faithful.*
– *I want to be unfaithful and use condoms with you, too – just in case I catch an infection and bring it back home.*
– *It's a good idea, just in case either of us is unfaithful.*
– *I trust you and hope you really trust me. If we use condoms routinely, you'll have more peace of mind and feel safer (just in case you don't really trust me but don't know how to tell me).*
– *I'd like us to use them so I can relax and feel that you feel safer, with me.*
❖ Should you make an absolute promise to remain faithful to each other and be honest, *before* either of you is unfaithful? This also gives you the chance to get your relationship back on course and avoid the so-called *need* to be unfaithful and the associated emotional hurt and pain.
❖ Should you go for a full STI check-up together, realise the implications of unfaithfulness and have an equal fear of the other's potential of being unfaithful. Then do you let that fear keep you faithful to your partner because of how you would feel if they were unfaithful to you and put your health at risk?
❖ Many people assume that it's OK to have unsafe sex with their regular partner but have safer sex with a casual partner.

* They think that using a condom is all the precaution necessary to keep their secret undiscovered.
* Not all sexually transmitted infections have instant signs or symptoms, but can ruin the good thing you had, when your regular partner realises they've been cheated, deceived and their health put at risk!
* Practise safer sex – ie:
(a) full STI check up before you have sex together. Re-testing after 3 months, if necessary.
(b) use a condom, routinely.
(c) be FAITHFUL or ABSTAIN *(NO SEX)*!
* Unfaithfulness is common, very unfair and brings nothing but misery when you're caught out.
* Being unfaithful includes casual sex with male or female sex workers *(prostitutes)*, casual gay or bisexual sex, having several regular partners or being involved in group sex *(orgy/swinging)*.

Remember:

* even the best condoms CAN fail.
* not all sexually transmitted infections show signs or give symptoms.
* practising safer sex routinely, could literally save your life.

What if we always have safer sex then want to have a baby?

* Each of you will want to know that you're safe from infection. The only sure way is for you and your partner to be fully tested at a GUM/STI Clinic *before* you have unprotected sex together.
* Again, you'll have to trust your partner isn't having sex outside your relationship – even if he/she uses a condom, you have no guarantee.
* After it's confirmed you can return to using condoms for protection throughout the pregnancy in case either of you has sex outside the relationship.
* Some men don't like to have sex with a pregnant woman. They find it impossible to remain faithful and stray towards someone else during this time – and make all kinds of excuses for their behaviour.
* If you're worried about having sex during pregnancy mention this to your Midwife or Doctor.
* It's usually safe for the woman (and your baby) to have sex well into pregnancy, so don't risk ruining a good relationship. Think *very* carefully before having sex elsewhere.
* Sex doesn't just mean penetration. There are many other ways to express close feelings and receive sexual pleasure and satisfaction.
* Potentially, it is serious for mother and baby to catch a sexually transmitted infection – and, of course, you'd be caught out.

* If you can't control your penis during your partner's pregnancy, you will almost certainly regret it later. And for what? A few minutes fun which you could still enjoy without penetration.
* Remember: respect your lady and you will enjoy the closeness of your family and new baby.

What about artificial insemination?

* Artificial insemination is where a female receives the sperm of a man without having sexual intercourse.
* Sperm donated to clinics specialising in this type of assisted fertility has, for many years, been tested for HIV – and some other infections.
* Sperm donated by a male friend for this purpose may put you at risk unless he has been fully tested for infection and counselled about the legal and emotional implications of donating sperm.
* Becoming pregnant through a one-night stand or other form of casual sex as a single parent *(or part of a lesbian couple bringing up a child together)* involves high-risk sex and you are strongly advised against it.

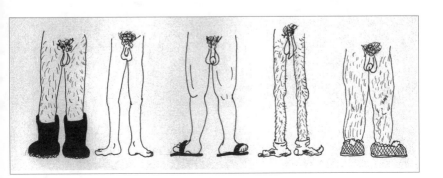

A sobering thought

- A woman is many times more likely to catch HIV from a man than a man is from a woman.
- Most men get HIV from one-night stands.
- Most women get HIV in long-term relationships.
- Many of these women find out that their partner has been unfaithful with another woman – although many find out it was with another man.
- A large number of men are closet *(secret)* bisexuals. They have sex with other men but are in denial. They don't consider themselves to be unfaithful to their female partner. They don't identify themselves as being gay or bisexual.
- They don't use safer sex correctly or sufficiently since many missed out on the information given throughout the gay community when HIV was first identified as an extremely serious infection.
- A large number of people *(heterosexual, homosexual and bisexual)* fail to enquire about the sexual history or infection status of a new partner before having sex.
- Having any STI increases your risk of contracting Hepatitis or HIV – and *vice-versa*.
- Hepatitis B virus can live for 2 weeks and Hepatitis C virus can live for 3 weeks in dried blood.
- 80% of the intravenous drug abusers *(junkies)* in the UK are said to be Hepatitis C positive.
- There is a vaccine against Hepatitis A and B – but NOT against Hepatitis C.
- Hepatitis B and C cause 82% of the world's liver cancer.
- By denying that you're at risk or failing to practise safer sex, you put your regular partner and, even perhaps your family, at risk – as well as yourself.
- You can only know your own sexual history, not that of your partner(s).

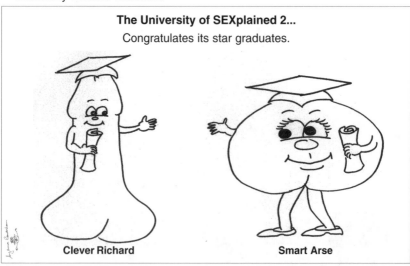

The University of SEXplained 2...
Congratulates its star graduates.

Clever Richard   **Smart Arse**

Some general points to remember

❖ You should: cover any broken or scabbed areas of skin or bleeding hang nails with water-proof plasters; or wear latex gloves for best protection from infection during foreplay.

❖ There's a risk of getting infection from unprotected oral sex. Germs can travel easily this way.

❖ If you get a sore throat after oral sex, don't be shy to tell the Doctor you see, so they can treat you properly.

❖ Unprotected anal sex is the highest risk form of sex.

❖ Having vaginal sex immediately after anal sex without changing to a new condom, is particularly dangerous. Germs from the bowel can pass easily into the vagina, womb and tubes unless you are meticulous about changing condoms.

❖ Vaginal sex before anal sex is safer if the condom cannot be changed.

❖ All sexually active people go to a GUM Clinic for a check up periodically.

❖ STIs are the most common infection caught after the common cold, so let's reduce the misery they cause and become more responsible.

Please note

❖ You may be at risk from Hepatitis B or C if you share cigarettes, spliffs, water pipes, crack pipes, *hubble-bubble;* or notes used to snort cocaine, with an infectious person.

❖ When kissing someone the risk of cross infection depends upon the state of both mouths – and whether there's blood in either person's saliva. In particular, a tiny amount of infected blood is sufficient to pass on the Hepatitis or Herpes virus.

But I can tell if she's a clean girl or dirty girl

❖ No, you can't. It's impossible to tell, just by looking, or talking to someone if they have a transmittable infection.

❖ Your nose, eyes or brain aren't capable of detecting hidden bacteria or viruses lurking in someone's genitalia.

You only have one life. It's easier to play a game of Russian roulette. At least with that the pain of dying is so quick you wouldn't feel it. Always use safer sexual protection.

Kat
Choreographer
& All Round Entertainer

Think twice!

❖ If you're a virgin, and your partner's also a virgin, you're having sex and contact with the germs of just one person.

❖ If you're a virgin and your first partner has had sex with, for example, 5 people, you're having sex and contact with the germs of a minimum of 6 people – *the other 5 plus your partner*.

❖ If you change partner *(now with your second partner)* and use the same theory, you have sex and contact with the germs of a minimum of 30 people *(their 5 partners and the 5 each of those have had)*.

❖ Change to your 3rd partner = a minimum of 155 people.

❖ Change again. Your 4th partner = a minimum of 780 people.

❖ 5th partner change = 3,905

❖ 6th partner change = 19,530

❖ 7th partner change = 97,655

❖ 8th partner change = 488,280

❖ 9th partner change = 2,441,405

❖ 10th partner change = 12,207,030

❖ **Plus, of course, all the people – all those *other* people – with whom they have had sex, too!**

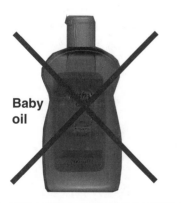

Baby oil

Which lubricants are safe to use with latex condoms and/or the female cap/diaphragm?

❖ Anything which is oil-based is unsafe to use with latex condoms and/or the female cap/diaphragm.

❖ Others are listed here:

VERY UNSAFE

❖ Everyday products which are considered UNSAFE to use with latex/rubber male condoms and the female cap/diaphragm.

1. Aromatherapy oils.
2. Margarine.
3. Butter.
4. Low-fat spreads.
5. Ice cream.
6. Salad cream/mayonnaise.
7. Cooking oils.
8. Suntan oil.
9. Lipstick.
10. Body oil.
11. Cold cream.
12. Baby oil.
13. Cocoa butter.
14. Massage oil.
15. Skin softener.
16. Hair conditioner.
17. Vaseline.
18. Petroleum Jelly.
19. Engine oil!
20. Cream.
21. Body paint.
22. Chocolate Spread/paint.
23. Some soaps *(oil based)*.

❖ Plus anything else which requires soap and water to wash them off your hands.

❖ **If there is *any* risk of viral hepatitis infection, saliva must not be used as a lubricant.**

UNSAFE

❖ Vaginal and rectal preparations which are considered UNSAFE to use with male latex/rubber condoms and the female cap/diaphragm.

1. Arachis oil enemas.
2. Baby oil.
3. Cyclogest.
4. Ecostatin.
5. Fungilin.
6. Gyno-Daktarin.
7. Gyno-Pevaryl.
8. Monistat.
9. Nizoral.
10. Nystan cream.
11. Petroleum Jelly.
12. Nystavescent.
13. Orthodienoestrol.
14. Orthogynest.
15. Pimafucin cream.
16. Rendel pessaries.
17. Sultrin.
18. Vaseline.
19. Witepsol-based suppositories.
20. Zinc and Castor oil.

❖ Plus anything else which requires soap and water to wash them off your hands.

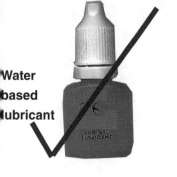

Water based lubricant

SAFE

❖ Vaginal and rectal preparations which are considered to be SAFE to use with male latex/rubber condoms or the female cap/diaphragm.

1. Aqueous enemas.
2. Aci-jel.
3. Boots lubricating jel.
4. Betadine.
5. Canesten.
6. Clotrimazole.
7. Delfen foam.
8. Delfen cream.
9. Double-check.
10. Durex Duragel.
11. Durex Duracreme.
12. Durex lubricating jel.
13. Durex Senselle.
14. Emko-foam.
15. Glycerin.
16. Gynol II.
17. Nyspes.
18. Nystan pessaries *(not cream)*.
19. Replens.
20. Staycept jelly.
21. Staycept pessaries.
22. Travogyn vaginal tablets.
23. Travogyn cream.
24. Two's company.
25. Aquagel.
26. K-Y Jelly.
27. Sutherland Jelly.
28. Wet.
29. Foreplay.
30. TLC.
31. Adonis.
32. Glyde Ultra.
33. Comfort.
34. Wet Fun flavours.
35. Cupid.
36. Sensual Succulents.

❖ Plus various other preparations which are available from specialist outlets but - always check first.

A healthy and well-mannered penis shall...........

1. Behave with dignity and allow his owner to have a wee in the morning, since his bladder is probably quite full after a night's sleep – despite his morning's glorious erection.

2. On a daily basis, change the underpants he lives within.

3. Be considerate of showing off his size and strength whilst in auto-erect mode within his owner's clothing and remain hidden from the view of others – except when invited out to play in private.

4. Ask his owner to treat him with respect during masturbation.

5. He'll have a wash at least once a day and clean away the smegma from around his glans (hood/helmet).

6. So he doesn't let himself or his owner down when encountering another's genitalia, be completely familiar with the look, feel and smell of condoms. He'll be competent at the skill of applying, using and, after ejaculation, removing them before he has his first sexual encounter.

7. Communicate with his owner and his testicular relatives on a regular basis. They must ensure they have no abnormal lumps, bumps, discharge or sores.

8. Be aware that condoms float, so used ones must be wrapped in a tissue and placed in a bin or other utensil for disposal, NOT flushed down the loo.

9. Treat himself to regular check ups at a GUM Clinic when sexually active.

10. Be aware of emergency contraception should his condom slip off during a sexual encounter with a female partner.

11. Behave with care and dignity when he finds a partner wanting him to visit, and encourage a return visit.

12. Ask permission to enter and clarify the situation before entry, rather than just assume it's alright; otherwise he may get a knock back and be rather embarrassed.

13. Stop, if his partner tells him to stop, or face the possibility of being charged with rape or sexual assault and going to prison!

He shall NOT...........

1. Embarrass his owner by becoming erect every time he senses an attractive person nearby. He'll learn to control these urges as he gets older or risk embarrassment by his continual desire to stand to attention.

2. Force himself or his presence onto or into anyone. He must only enter and exercise himself with the full and express consent of his partner.

3. Get trapped in trouser zips *(ouch)*!

4. Complain if he overdoes foreplay. His testicular accomplices may complain of an ache *(blue ball)* the next day. They won't be harmed, but this can be relieved by masturbation.

5. Worry about getting trapped inside his partner during sex, for he needs to be erect and strong to gain entry. He can pull out at any time. He'll return to his pre-erect size and softness after ejaculating, so he can slip out unharmed – but must not forget to hold his condom in place as he withdraws.

6. Even attempt to have sex with anyone who is under the legal age of consent in the country in which he is erect at the time.

7. Assume it's a green light to proceed to sex just because someone allows a certain amount of intimate foreplay.

8. Even think of having sex without wearing a condom to protect himself from invisible invading bugs or lurgy.

9. When wearing a condom, he'll withdraw before he goes limp after ejaculation when wearing a condom; otherwise it's likely to remain inside his partner, rendering its use ineffective. In other words, he must withdraw whilst still hard, holding the condom in place as he does so, to ensure that it doesn't get left inside his partner.

10. Have sex if he fears he might have an infection. He should get thoroughly checked up by the GUM Clinic, *before* he resumes sexual activity.

11. Rub himself up, down or around his partner's genitalia without wearing a condom.

12. Assume that a female partner is using birth control, but wear a condom *at all times* when encountering female genitalia.

13. The only exception is if his owner is fully prepared for the consequences of unplanned pregnancy and he has a healthy bank balance to support his partner and any future offspring.

13. Continue if he senses that his condom has slipped off or down. He must stop and reconsider the situation. Emergency Contraception might be advisable.

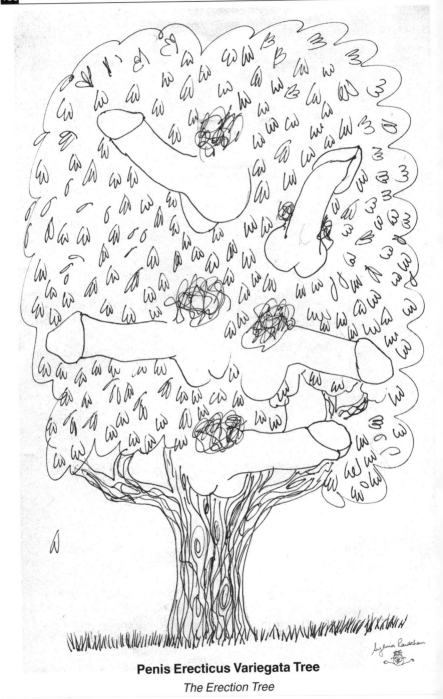

Penis Erecticus Variegata Tree

The Erection Tree

Identification

❖ It's wise to carry photographic ID *(identification)* as proof of your age and to prevent any embarrassing moments when trying to gain entry to clubs – especially if you look younger than your age.

Clothing

❖ No-one has the right to touch you without permission. However much you may dislike it, you'll be judged by the clothes you wear.

❖ It can be dangerous to try to be more grown up than your years, to tease or act provocatively, just to experience adult life!

❖ Your self-confidence will grow with age and experience but it's wise to wear clothes in which you feel comfortable, especially in relation to the comments or actions you'll provoke.

❖ You may want to dress provocatively – eg. in skin-tight clothes – to attract others, but beware of the non-verbal signals you give to others.

❖ Do wear underwear, even if you do want to conceal your *panty lines,* otherwise you will invite trouble.

❖ Don't make the mistake of thinking *an attack couldn't happen to me*, it could and it can.

❖ Be perfectly clear about the behaviour you will or won't allow.

❖ Carry an attack alarm in your handbag and don't be afraid to use it, if you feel frightened or need help.

Theft and pickpockets

❖ Don't flash your cash!

❖ Pickpockets abound. Nightclubs are no safer than crowded tube trains when it comes to theft.

❖ Be particularly careful when carrying cash and credit cards. You may be watched when, after use, you return them to your bag or pocket.

❖ Don't carry more money or credit cards than you need to use at any one time.

❖ Don't carry a chequebook. Just carry one or two cheques. Keep them away from your cheque-card.

❖ Always try to keep enough money for a cab fare home and if necessary keep this in a separate place. Even if you go out with friends, you may find you want to leave before or after them and to have the cab fare handy may save your life.

❖ It's always much safer to go to and leave a club or party in a group.

❖ It's safer to take a licensed cab than risk walking alone at night. **NEVER** accept a lift from a stranger.

❖ Only use a *recognised* mini-cab company.

❖ If you can't afford to get home, you can't afford to go out!

Mobile phones and handbags

❖ Beware of someone who gives you a mobile phone number – but no land line number. Maybe they live with someone or it may simply be a precaution since they don't know *you*. If in doubt, wonder why, then ask!

❖ Take care of *your* mobile phone. Don't leave it lying around while you go to dance. Don't leave it in your coat pocket in a cloakroom.

❖ Avoid handbags if possible. Use a *bum bag/belt bag* or something else you can wear while dancing.

❖ For security reasons, remove combs, nail files, sprays etc. from your handbag before entering a club – or leave them at home – since they are considered potential weapons. If you don't, the door supervisor may confiscate them until you leave the club.

❖ Don't put your handbag on the floor or by your feet when standing in a crowd having a drink; or while dancing.

❖ Don't put your handbag by your side when seated unless it's zipped up or closed properly.

❖ Keep the closed end of the zip or flap nearest your front and keep the bag closely attached to you in some way, *at all times*.

❖ Even when it's over your shoulder, in your hand or on the floor by your feet, a clever pickpocket can take contents from it without you even feeling their presence!

Men hunt in packs

❖ Go to a club or a party in a crowd and leave with that crowd. NEVER go off alone with a stranger – or someone you've been chatting to all evening. He/she is still a stranger.

❖ If you notice a group of young men watching you with your friends before you go to dance, be particularly careful not to leave your drink where it could be 'spiked' *(have a drug slipped into it without you knowing)*.

❖ When you flirt or tease, make sure you don't lead a man on – unless you're prepared for the consequences.

❖ Avoid being over friendly, since you may give off the wrong signals. It could lead to trouble you may not be able to handle.

Lone danger

❖ Beware of the attention of lone men and don't become isolated from your friends.

❖ Bring anyone or anything you feel uncomfortable about to the attention of the club's security staff. They should be able to help.

Casual sex

❖ Today, casual sex is more dangerous. Medical advances and expensive treatments don't necessarily provide a cure for all infections passed on through casual sex.

❖ If you buy condoms from a vending machine in a club, make sure they're still *in date* and that they're not gimmick condoms.

❖ Check for the British Standard kitemark, the CE or EN600 mark on the packet or understand the standard to which they are made.

❖ It's impossible to know someone's sexual history or whether they have a sexually transmitted infection in just one evening.

❖ Think of tomorrow, not just the moment! Look after yourself and if they care about you at all, they'll wait – if they won't wait, then you've lost nothing!

❖ Don't put yourself at risk for the sake of a thrill or someone else's ego.

❖ If you decide to have casual sex make sure you use a condom and other protection correctly, especially if you're just giving or receiving oral sex *(blow job)*.

Look after each other better

❖ If you see your female friends OR your male friends drunk or otherwise *under the weather* whilst out clubbing, look out for their safety – not just your own. In this state they are vulnerable and a potential victim of crime. By keeping a watchful eye on them, you could prevent them from harm.

Accepting a lift

❖ Don't accept a lift if you feel uncomfortable, particularly if the driver has been drinking alcohol, or taking drugs.

❖ When you get into someone's car, you're entering their territory. You can't get out when you want – the driver will be in control.

❖ You won't know how well they can drive but your life may well depend on it.

Set a new trend.

Celibacy is sexy.

But if you're not sexy – make <u>sure</u> you're safe.

Leila
Sex Worker of the Year '98

Mini-cabs

❖ If you're uncomfortable about someone who's offering you a lift home, get a cab home.

❖ Phone for a licensed, on duty and properly insured, identifiable cabdriver, from a legitimate company. Always ask for – and write down – the name of the driver and their cab driver's ID number.

❖ Ask for a pre-arranged code word to identify them further, when they arrive.

❖ Wait in a well lit place with someone else – if possible.

❖ Don't approach him/her first. When the driver approaches, ask him/her to give his/her name. Don't simply ask: *are you eg. John Smith*. A genuine cabbie won't mind at all.

❖ Ask to see their photographic ID.

❖ *Touts* often offer to get young women cabs. These are often unlicensed and sometimes operated by criminal gangs for the purpose of gaining money, sex – or both – from female groups or single passengers.

❖ Many criminals evade police checks and work as *pirate cabbies* – often without insurance.

❖ Even if it's late and you have to wait for a cab, NEVER take a *pirate cab*. Don't accept identification in the form of a business card. Anyone can have business cards. They don't prove a thing!

❖ Some *pirate cabbies* clock off from a shift with a legitimate firm and work for themselves for a few hours, to avoid paying commission to their employer.

❖ A *pirate cabbie* won't be in regular radio contact with his base, even if they've got a radio in their car, with an extra arial. This is to trick you into thinking they're genuine.

❖ Don't assume that because a door supervisor *(bouncer)* hails you a cab, you'll be safe – and don't take his/her word for it that you'll be OK. He doesn't know that for sure.

Advice when entering someone's home for the first time

❖ Being alone with someone for the first time may be exciting but it can also make you feel a little nervous. It is sensible, therefore, to be cautious. Ensure that you tell someone where you're going and with whom. Arrange to call this friend to *check in* when you arrive and as you leave – or by an agreed time. If your friend doesn't hear from you by the agreed time, they can then decide whether or not to contact the Police and ask them to check up on your safety.

❖ A genuine friend won't mind how many precautions you take.

❖ When you arrive:

(a) check whether anyone else is there – especially if you expect to be alone with your host.

(b) make a mental note of the layout when you arrive.

(c) check your exit routes in case of fire or fear.

(d) let your host know that someone is waiting to hear from you, knows where you are and who you're with, by name. Your host now knows that someone else is looking out for your safety.

(e) observe your surroundings to ensure it's their home or whether it's a place used for seduction/sex!

(f) if you feel uncomfortable, make an excuse and leave quickly.

(g) call to check in – as pre-arranged.

Being alone with strangers

❖ Be especially careful if you invite a stranger into your home. NEVER give your address to someone you've just met – however charming he/she may seem. Get to know and trust them.

❖ Love yourself enough to take time to get to know a person on neutral territory *(out in public)* – eg. a cafe, with friends etc.

❖ It's safer, but not foolproof, if they're already known to someone you know well, who can vouch for their good character.

❖ NEVER invite a stranger into your home, even for coffee, until you feel safe and secure with them.

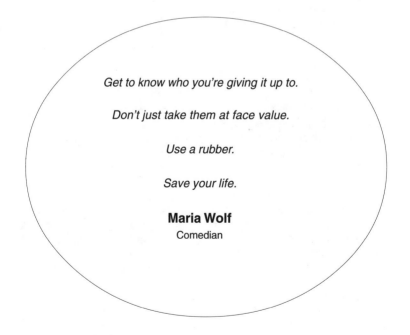

Get to know who you're giving it up to.

Don't just take them at face value.

Use a rubber.

Save your life.

Maria Wolf
Comedian

Safer Dating and Clubbing SEXplained...®

Date Rape

❖ Be aware of *date rape* drugs.

❖ A certain type of man may plan to rape *(force someone to have sex without consent)* before they leave home, and take *date rape* drugs with them.

❖ Stranger rape, when the attacker is unknown to the victim, is what most people associate with rape.

❖ Date rape is when someone you know and feel you can trust, rapes you.

❖ Date rape and acquaintance rape *(not a stranger but not someone you know well)* is far more common than *stranger rape*.

❖ Men *(gay or straight)* are also at risk of rape and sexual assault.

❖ Drugs such as *roofies, (Rohypnol)* or another type of mind-altering drug, are slipped into your drink.

❖ In the dark, you'll be unaware of any change in the colour or taste of your drink. The change of colour – which shows blue in a light coloured drink – takes 20 minutes. By which time, you'll probably have consumed it, anyway.

❖ Their method of operation is to lead you away to a lonely corner – eg. toilet or car park – or even perhaps go home with you or invite you to their place.

❖ The drugs make you fall asleep. You could be raped and, because you'd be so sleepy, you wouldn't remember much about the incident *(or them)*. The drugs have an amnesic *(loss of memory)* effect. You'd wake up to realise something's not right and may feel that you've been raped.

❖ Some rapists even wear a condom, in an attempt to conceal *(hide)* evidence.

❖ If you see anyone slip something into a drink, you MUST first report it to the nightclub security AND the Police. If they suspect rape, they will arrange for a medical examination, emergency contraception and STI advice and check up as soon as possible.

❖ Even if you don't want an examination or aren't sure what happened but feel you may have been raped, it's important to get to the Police within 24 hours *(or as soon as possible)* after feeling odd *(or as if you've been raped)* to have a special blood or urine test. This will be used as evidence and will help the Police find your attacker.

Rape

❖ There are three types of rapist:

(a) stranger rapist.

(b) acquaintance rapist.

(c) date rapist.

❖ It's an alarming fact that more rapes are carried out by men known to their victims than by strangers.

❖ Usually, rapists are unpredictable bullies of any shape, size, colour or creed.

❖ Many are good looking, likeable and often, charming men. Indeed they may be the last person you'd think would ever need to rape a woman.

❖ Rape has little to do with sex. It has far more to do with exerting power and control over another person.

❖ They *get off* on terrorising their victim.

❖ Some don't accept they've done anything wrong – and spend years in denial. Many are very devious *conmen*.

❖ Many excuse their behaviour by saying that their victim was 'up for it' *(ready for sex)* – ie. by their suggestive clothing or actions – and cried rape after the event.

❖ Some men are not confident about their sexuality. They may even believe it's their *right* to have sex with someone who flirts innocently with them, goes out for a meal or spends time alone with them.

❖ They don't stop to think how they would feel if their mother, sister or even their son or daughter was the victim.

❖ **Every victim has a mother – as does every attacker.**

❖ Few men are rapists. But **any man could rape** and **any woman could be raped**.

❖ **Male rape** happens too. Men need to be equally aware. No matter how big and strong you are, you'd be weak against a gang intent on rape.

❖ Female or male – no one has the right to force another person to do ANYTHING against their will.

❖ Sadly, in some inner city areas, gang rape – rape by more than one man – appears to be increasing, so be vigilant.

What to do

❖ If you're ever sexually assaulted or raped, DO tell the Police.

❖ Remember, however terrified you may be, your attacker WILL strike again. He *could* kill his next victim. An attacker must be caught and stopped. Give the Police all they need – eg. clothing, bedding, towels etc. used during or straight after the incident – as soon as possible. This will help secure a conviction and other people will be safe from your attacker.

❖ Note: It is a serious offence to accuse someone of rape without justification.

Are there any organisations around to help men with a history of violence?

❖ There are a few excellent organisations. They specialise in helping men who have a history of violence either towards their partner or who hate women, despite an outward display of adulation.

❖ Whatever excuse you use for losing your temper, which leads to violence – *eg. alcohol, drugs, history of abuse or simply something someone does to upset you*, you should NEVER take your anger out on others.

❖ You may think you've got to appear big and tough but remember, it takes a big man to admit he has problems and a bigger man to seek help in dealing with them.

❖ Be brave, pick up the phone and get help before it's too late.

❖ *For further information on violence see page 182-183.*

Swapping addresses or phone numbers

❖ Don't give your address or phone number to someone you don't know without thinking of the consequences.

❖ Make sure you're not overheard when giving out details in public – eg. shop, club, etc. In the wrong hands, your address and telephone number could be used to commit crime – either in your name (!) or with *you* as a victim of crime.

Don't accept things from strangers or casual acquaintances

It is unwise to accept the following from strangers:

❖ **A drink.** It may be laced *(mixed)* with a *date rape drug* or other drug.

❖ **Chewing gum.** It may be laced with LSD/speed.

❖ **Ecstacy.** It may be laced with heroin.

❖ **Cigarettes (*or spliffs* or *joints*).** They may be laced with cocaine and/or heroin.

❖ **Viagra.** Unless you're being treated for impotence, it may seriously affect your erectile function. It MUST only be used under medical supervision since it interacts badly with some other drugs and could be fatal.

You shouldn't just be thinking about having sex, but about making love with someone you seriously care about.

Gary Cameron
Actor

Drink, drugs and fights

- ❖ Unprotected sex is often a consequence of too much alcohol – so don't have too much – or mix types of alcohol. Getting drunk means you're likely to take more risks and go home with someone to whom you'd not normally be attracted.

- ❖ When a person is under the influence of drink, drugs or both, they lose their inhibitions, and common sense. They often *get carried away* sexually – taking more risks. They then worry about pregnancy and/or infection the next day!

- ❖ Don't leave your drink at a table or at the bar when you go to dance.

- ❖ It's safer to drink from a can or bottle.

- ❖ Keep your drink with you at ALL times so it can't be 'spiked' *(a drug slipped into it without you realising).* Someone may do this for 'fun' but it is a criminal offence. Also, they are unlikely to know your medical history or whether you are taking any medication. They could find themselves facing serious criminal charges – for example, murder, attempted murder or manslaughter if you react seriously to the combination and collapse.

- ❖ In addition – alcohol mixed with some drugs can cause serious complications – and could be fatal.

- ❖ So, if you put your drink down or leave it – even with a friend – don't touch it again. Buy a new drink from the bar.

- ❖ If you're involved in a fight and blood is drawn, assume you're at risk of catching **hepatitis** and seek medical advice within 24 hours.

Five minutes of fun isn't worth a lifetime of regret.

Kat
Choreographer
& All Round Entertainer

When to contact the Police

Contact the Police:

❖ if you're particularly frightened or uncomfortable about a situation – or by a particular person. They may already know the person in connection with similar or worse things. Even if they don't, they should be aware of people who make others frightened.

❖ Remember: the Police can't do anything to help the public, without information.

Will I have to make a formal complaint?

❖ No, you won't have to make a formal complaint. You can tell them what's happened and let them guide you from there.

❖ Even if you make an allegation against someone – but don't want to proceed with a charge against them – if you have clear reasons for not wanting to proceed, the Police won't think you're wasting their time.

❖ It's not being silly or making a fuss about nothing.

❖ You should always trust your instincts.

Why is it so important to contact the Police?

It's important to contact the Police for several reasons:

❖ harassment is a crime and is against the Law. The Law is there to protect you – stand firm and use it to protect yourself.

❖ most bullies are basically cowards and if they are not stopped they will continue to frighten more victims.

❖ sometimes, just realising that a victim refuses to be bullied any more – even if it means they have asked the Police to help them – the bully stops his disgraceful behaviour.

❖ you may also need support from friends or family but don't let a bully – of any description – get away with intimidating you.

I'm not being harassed but I want the Police to know about something. I don't want to give them my name, so what can I do?

❖ You can ring *Crimestoppers* on their *freephone* number 0800 555 111 (UK)

❖ You don't need to give your name.

❖ Your call could help to protect other people.

❖ Your call could prevent a crime.

❖ You could receive a cash reward.

People with physical or mental disability

❖ Don't *walk on the other side* because any one of us could become disabled.

❖ The information provided in this book is as much for able bodied as it is for people with a physical or mental disability.

❖ Just because someone is disabled or has learning difficulties doesn't, of course, preclude them from wanting to be loved emotionally and physically.

❖ Those of us who are fortunate enough to be able bodied should stop to think for a minute. *How would I feel if I was less able bodied or if I had learning difficulties?*

❖ If you know someone like this, do what you can to help him/her to have an enjoyable social life.

❖ It's harder to find nightclubs, restaurants etc. with suitable provision for wheelchairs but they do exist and there's an increasing amount of information and support available from various organisations.

❖ Girls with certain learning difficulties – eg. Down's syndrome – often start their periods slightly earlier than usual and may appear to be less inhibited sexually.

❖ They are equally at risk of unplanned pregnancy, or sexually transmitted infections.

❖ BUT they are often less able to give their informed consent to have sex.

❖ Sometimes, people who've suffered a severe head injury – eg. from a car crash or boxing accident – behave in a way which is sexually inappropriate. This needs to be understood by friends and family. They may need gentle help to understand and re-learn how to behave with other people.

❖ Young men with spinal injuries who are unable to get an erection need to discuss their difficulties with their doctor. Various products are available to help all forms of impotence.

❖ *For further information on organisations for less able bodied people and people with learning difficulties see page 182.*

*Life's full of risks but an accident could happen to any of us.
It could happen to you. It could happen to me.
Stick within safe limits. Take one step at a time.
Don't disrespect someone less able.
How would you feel if that person was you.*

Jason Matthews
Commonwealth
Middleweight Boxing Champion 1999

*Be careful
or it could get embarrassing if you
get a little itch or discharge
after sex.*

*You might bump in to someone you
know at the clinic!*

Eddie Nestor
Actor/Comedian

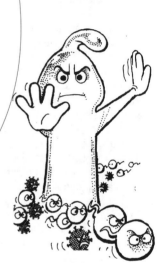

Remember:
barrier protection – prevents infection

*When the prick is hard,
the brain is in the balls.
So for God's sake, wear a condom.*
Cynthia Payne
1998

Is there anything I should be aware of?

* GUM is the new name for an STI Clinic.
* Previously, these were known as special, VD or nicknamed 'clap' clinics.
* Usually GUM Clinics are open Monday to Friday, from 9am to 5pm.
* Ring your local hospital to check their opening times and whether they run an appointment system, a *walk-in* clinic – or both services.
* You will be seen on the day you decide to attend.
* You don't need to be referred to this clinic by your GP. You can walk in and ask to be seen.
* Sometimes you may have to wait if they are very busy. They diagnose some test results while you wait. This takes time but you'll be given the correct treatment for your specific infection, FREE OF CHARGE.
* Some have a special *fast lane* or prioritised and speedy walk-in service for male and female sex workers *(also known as working women/men, or prostitutes)*.

What else is available?

* All counselling and medication is provided FREE OF CHARGE.
* If you're on *income support* your fares will be reimbursed.
* Hepatitis B vaccination is available. Usually, it's 3 injections over 7 months.
* Some GUM/STI Clinics provide Emergency Contraceptive pills up to 72 hours after unprotected sex.

* Normally, emergency IUD/IUCDs are not inserted in GUM/STI clinics. However, they may be willing to refer you to a Family Planning Clinic.
* If you have a pelvic infection at the time, a coil/IUCD is not advisable.
* GUM Clinics do cervical smear tests. If any abnormalities are found, further tests and treatment can also be done quickly and accurately.

Is everything confidential?

* By Law, their service must be confidential.
* They won't tell you what your partner has, nor will they tell your partner what you have – unless you request their help and intervention.
* They won't inform your GP of anything unless you give permission.

If they keep notes on me, what information do they need?

* They will ask you for:
  – a name.
  – date of birth.
  – contact address.
* The details *should* be your own – but this is not essential. You can make up a name.
* The name and date of birth you give are used purely for internal administration and filing.
* If you give a false name/address you'll need to remember it for future visits to the clinic – without the correct details they won't find your notes quickly and/or easily.

Who will I see?

❖ Doctors, Nurses and clerical staff; and health advisors explain about each infection and help you understand what has to be done to make you well again.

❖ A psychosexual counsellor *(to talk sexual problems through)* often works in the GUM/STI clinic.

How can I help the staff?

To ensure better results:

❖ MEN can help by not passing urine for 3 - 4 hours before any swabs or specimens are taken.

❖ WOMEN can help by working out in advance the date of the first day of your last period.

❖ It's OK to attend when you have a period but the staff are unlikely to do a smear test or colposcopy – and may ask you to return. However other tests can be carried out.

What's a contact slip and why do some people get one?

❖ A contact slip is a specially coded piece of paper, which tells another Doctor which specific infection(s) should be checked.

❖ If you're given a contact slip they will ask you to give it to your sexual partner(s).

❖ They can then take it into any GUM/STI clinic in the country for examination and receive the appropriate treatment.

❖ Following the recommended treatment is the best way you can help the doctors and avoid re-infection.

Can I have an HIV test at a GUM/STI clinic?

❖ Totally confidential HIV counselling and testing are available.

❖ Nowadays, same day HIV test results are available by appointment at many clinics.

❖ Treatment is available for those who are *HIV antibody positive* with referral to other hospital departments, including dental, community and social care.

❖ Some clinics give general test results over the phone – but NOT HIV test results.

General information

❖ Don't be shy. Answer all questions openly and honestly. You won't shock anyone working in a GUM/STI clinic.

❖ Most infections are treatable. If you delay treatment because of embarrassment, the problem could get worse. So, go early and get a problem sorted out.

❖ If you think you have an infection, NEVER take a friend's medication or some that you see lying around. It could make the problem worse.

❖ Visit the clinic for correct diagnosis and in date medication for what you HAVE got.

❖ If you notice any abnormal lumps, bumps, blisters or discharge, particularly in your genital area, get it checked.

❖ Everyone should have a check up, from time to time.

❖ Germs can spread genitally *(down below)* or orally *(by mouth)* so – safer oral and penetrative sex is vital.

❖ Remember: having a sexually transmitted infection increases your risk of contracting HIV or HEPATITIS.

❖ Many STIs which cause open wounds, are highly infectious. Therefore, when treating an open wound or sore from a STI you must avoid cross infection, either to a different area of your own body or to the body of someone else.

❖ Wear disposable latex gloves when treating a wet or oozing wound/sore.

❖ Dispose of any soiled dressings in a plastic bag. Wrap or seal the bag, before throwing it out with the rubbish.

❖ Alternatively, ask a qualified nurse to teach you how to change a dressing, using an aseptic or no-touch technique.

❖ Do all you can to prevent cross infection. Don't put others at risk.

❖ To prevent cross infection/ contamination, always wash your hands with soap and hot water after passing urine, opening your bowels, touching your own or anyone else's genitalia, or changing a baby's nappy – especially if you'll be preparing food.

❖ You don't always receive immunity against future infection by having an infection once.

❖ It's possible to get some sexually transmitted infections more than once, so protect yourself at all times.

Word Search

T	E	A	S	E	B	V	A	G	I	N	A	L	M	E	V	R	T	B
P	E	T	T	I	N	G	D	I	N	F	E	C	T	I	O	N	Z	R
A	P	D	P	E	R	I	O	D	S	E	X	U	A	L	I	T	Y	E
B	G	T	A	D	P	O	L	E	S	L	A	W	P	V	C	A	H	A
G	H	A	E	P	U	B	E	R	T	Y	E	S	P	I	E	I	Y	S
H	Y	G	I	E	N	E	S	E	X	D	H	R	U	R	P	L	D	T
K	M	R	D	W	Q	E	C	T	O	P	I	C	B	G	R	L	R	S
L	F	E	R	T	I	L	E	M	U	C	U	S	I	I	O	Y	O	A
T	A	B	U	S	E	P	N	O	H	S	T	W	C	N	S	S	C	R
W	E	I	G	H	T	R	C	M	N	M	I	D	E	H	T	P	E	M
O	R	I	S	T	E	E	E	C	T	O	P	I	C	T	A	E	L	P
P	E	N	I	S	S	G	A	E	I	K	J	E	W	S	T	R	E	I
A	C	O	D	G	T	N	B	R	N	I	G	T	I	T	E	M	G	T
R	T	R	R	R	I	A	R	V	F	N	P	I	B	E	R	T	A	E
E	I	G	E	O	C	N	Y	I	E	G	E	N	I	T	A	L	R	B
N	O	A	A	I	L	T	O	X	R	E	F	G	A	Y	G	O	O	I
T	N	S	M	N	E	M	A	S	T	U	R	B	A	T	E	V	U	T
H	Y	M	E	N	V	E	C	L	I	T	O	R	I	S	C	E	S	E
C	L	O	T	H	E	S	C	O	L	P	O	S	C	O	P	Y	A	S
H	E	A	L	T	H	Y	S	M	E	A	R	T	E	S	T	S	L	X

- healthy
- puberty
- adolescence
- fertile
- mucus
- periods
- virgin
- love
- bites
- armpit
- groin
- wet
- dream
- discharge
- vaginal
- ectopic * 2
- sex
- cervix
- sexuality

- parent
- smoking
- drugs
- dieting
- weight
- public
- gay
- sperm
- voice
- erection
- penis
- abuse
- tease
- testicle
- masturbation
- genital
- tadpoles
- hydrocele
- prostate

- clothes
- infection
- pregnant
- infertile
- hygiene
- arousal
- no
- yes
- law
- clitoris
- petting
- hymen
- smear
- test
- colposcopy
- orgasm
- breasts

Answers on page 181.

Language and Respect

❖ People are judged mostly by their language. You'll want to be respected by others but *to get respect you have to give respect*.

❖ It's not what you say, it's how you say it.

❖ *Loud mouths* try to show off and use bad language – most people don't like *loud mouths*!

❖ Your language tells your listener a lot about you. Using disrespectful terms can have the opposite effect from what you want – it's one sure way to LOSE other people's respect!

❖ How would you feel about someone if you heard them describe your mother, sister, partner or friend in disrespectful terms - then think about the language you use.

❖ Discuss the following provocative list of alternative words with your friends and then decide what types of people use these words.

Sexual intercourse:

❖ make love
❖ have sex
❖ screw
❖ fuck
❖ bonk
❖ rootle
❖ shaft
❖ root
❖ play
❖ party
❖ sex-up
❖ sex
❖ do it
❖ jucky jam your beef
❖ shag
❖ quickie
❖ a poke
❖ dip the wick
❖ porking
❖ frig
❖ freak
❖ dig out
❖ whack
❖ oats
❖ piece
❖ sleep together
❖ shaft
❖ jiggy jiggy
❖ slam it
❖ grind
❖ wynd
❖ bash the gash
❖ bedroom stabbing
❖ humping
❖ nookie
❖ tomming
❖ shunt
❖ sink the sub
❖ hide the ferret
❖ poke the hole
❖ rumpy pumpy
❖ hide the sausage
❖ sail yer semen
❖ parting meaty gates
❖ shrimp
❖ pole vaulting
❖ oil change
❖ drill
❖ cock-up
❖ boompsing
❖ give him/her one
❖ leg over
❖ can I plant my dipstick in your garden?
❖ can I put my submarine in your harbour?
❖ I'd like to plant some seed in your garden
❖ can I hide my mole in your hole?
❖ rub out your crease

Vagina

- ❖ vag
- ❖ cunt
- ❖ pum-pum
- ❖ love tunnel
- ❖ punanny
- ❖ punny
- ❖ fanny (UK)
- ❖ pearly gates
- ❖ tunnel of love
- ❖ pussy
- ❖ pussy hole
- ❖ hole
- ❖ twat
- ❖ minge
- ❖ pleasure hole
- ❖ meat hole
- ❖ fatty
- ❖ fridge
- ❖ beaver
- ❖ slit
- ❖ coal hole
- ❖ G-spot
- ❖ jammy dodger
- ❖ crack
- ❖ beef
- ❖ cho cho
- ❖ veggie
- ❖ Mary

External genitalia

- ❖ vulva
- ❖ Miss Min
- ❖ pussy
- ❖ muff
- ❖ crotch
- ❖ boxcrutch
- ❖ buff
- ❖ minge
- ❖ clit
- ❖ hairy meat-pie
- ❖ beef curtains
- ❖ lips
- ❖ slot
- ❖ piss-flaps

Breasts

- ❖ tits
- ❖ top bollocks
- ❖ melons
- ❖ jugs
- ❖ boobs
- ❖ knockers
- ❖ titties
- ❖ pleasure domes
- ❖ bosoms
- ❖ bazookas
- ❖ mammaries
- ❖ milkbar
- ❖ bra-buster
- ❖ d-cups
- ❖ double Ds
- ❖ door stoppers
- ❖ water melons
- ❖ fried eggs
- ❖ poached eggs
- ❖ pancakes
- ❖ jumbos

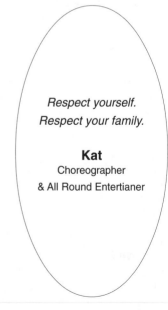

Respect yourself.
Respect your family.

Kat
Choreographer
& All Round Entertianer

Oral sex

- ❖ felattio
- ❖ cunnilingus
- ❖ a Monica
- ❖ fur burger
- ❖ muff diving
- ❖ 69
- ❖ soixante-neuf
- ❖ lick his pole
- ❖ blow job (BJ)
- ❖ give head
- ❖ lick
- ❖ go down
- ❖ massage
- ❖ shine/r
- ❖ grow at the beaver
- ❖ boof Danny sex
- ❖ suck
- ❖ foreplay
- ❖ mega-bite
- ❖ giga-bite
- ❖ swallow
- ❖ French roll wash
- ❖ rinse out
- ❖ gobble
- ❖ pearl diving
- ❖ going downtown

Penis

- ❖ willy
- ❖ trunchoen
- ❖ pole
- ❖ John Thomas
- ❖ Hercules
- ❖ love muscle
- ❖ prick
- ❖ pork sword
- ❖ shaft
- ❖ meat
- ❖ angle grinder
- ❖ cock
- ❖ old man
- ❖ bone
- ❖ two peas and a maggot
- ❖ meat and two veg
- ❖ baton
- ❖ knob
- ❖ well endowed
- ❖ love stick
- ❖ pyjma python
- ❖ trouser snake
- ❖ banana
- ❖ torpedo
- ❖ licorice stick
- ❖ member
- ❖ third leg
- ❖ todger
- ❖ jammy todger
- ❖ frankfurter
- ❖ buzz stick
- ❖ tackle
- ❖ wood
- ❖ hood
- ❖ boy
- ❖ plonker
- ❖ Dick
- ❖ totem pole
- ❖ benu Dick
- ❖ manhood
- ❖ deadly laser
- ❖ Percy
- ❖ love laser
- ❖ thing
- ❖ Mr Johnson

SEXplained...® List of Alternative Words

Erection

- boner
- hard-on
- bone-on
- stiffy
- rock-hard
- attention seeker
- standing to attention
- rampant pork sword
- rifle
- big Ben
- Albert
- carrot
- flag pole
- cock-up
- cucumber
- Eiffel Tower
- cock stand
- stiffner
- a serious Johnson

Masturbate

- safe sex
- wank
- DIY
- play with yourself
- hand relief
- visit Miss Palmer
- beat the meat
- beat the monkey
- bash the pole
- bash the todger
- spank the monkey
- love for one
- solo sex
- self sex
- breast releif
- five knuckle shuffle
- J Arthur
- toss off
- waz
- Tommy tank
- choke yer chicken
- slap yer granny
- slap the salami
- yank yer plank
- palming
- pray to the urinal
- handy Andy
- stroke the ferret
- frankspurter
- four finger shuffle
- emission
- back yer wrist
- jerk off
- slap your wrist
- have a pully
- say hello to the 5-fingered widow
- howl at the moon

Bisexual

- AC/DC
- swings both ways

Homosexual

- gay
- poof
- faggot
- tosser
- shirt lifter
- homo
- queer
- queen
- tart
- sads
- bum basher
- bottoms up
- bugger
- fairy
- fanny (USA)
- poofta
- queenie
- rent boy
- navy cake
- bent as a ten bob note
- bent
- dyke
- butch
- lesbo
- glads

Trans-sexual/transvestitie

- ❖ he, she, it
- ❖ heshe
- ❖ feMale
- ❖ heMale
- ❖ it
- ❖ cross dresser

- ❖ A lot of these words display discrimination against homo-sexuals.
- ❖ How do you think your best friend, brother or sister would feel about you if s/he heard you talking like this, when they were hoping to confide in you that *they* are homosexual or bisexual?
- ❖ You'd probably lose their close friendship and not know why. The damage could prove to be too much for your broken friendship to repair.

Terms for sexually experienced female

- ❖ whore
- ❖ slag
- ❖ tart
- ❖ slapper
- ❖ Tom
- ❖ slut
- ❖ scumbag
- ❖ bike
- ❖ losh
- ❖ hag
- ❖ bitch
- ❖ dirty little rooter
- ❖ hooker
- ❖ ripper
- ❖ shosher
- ❖ shortie
- ❖ bird
- ❖ stopout
- ❖ pussy whore
- ❖ sketz
- ❖ bint
- ❖ mort
- ❖ easy
- ❖ loose
- ❖ 'b' with an itch
- ❖ prostitute
- ❖ brass
- ❖ nympho (nymphomaniac)
- ❖ matress
- ❖ cunt
- ❖ bimbo
- ❖ hussy
- ❖ dirty matress
- ❖ dirty gutter
- ❖ charlatan
- ❖ come around
- ❖ prick teaser
- ❖ scrubber
- ❖ old boot
- ❖ cow
- ❖ jezebel

- ❖ None of these words or phrases are respectful to women. Why?

Terms for sexually experienced male

* Jack the lad
* one of the boys/lads
* player
* gigolo
* dirty old git
* randy sod
* male slag
* playboy
* Casanova
* lucky bastard
* tart
* sperm doner
* super sperm
* sperm banker
* hoe
* dog
* earth mover
* goodun
* darg
* rooster
* old lad
* old dog
* male whore
* Virtually all these words give the opposite image to the words used for sexually experienced women. That's neither right, not fair – why?
* You may know different words for some or all of these. Many display disrespect. Which are they and why are they disrespectful?
* Before YOU use these words, which may discriminate towards other people, think for a moment about how YOU would feel if YOU were called any of these names – even in fun.

Some men are stupid.

Their excuse for not wearing a condom is that they don't want their Dick to look like a miniature bank rubber!

Glaz Campbell
Comedian

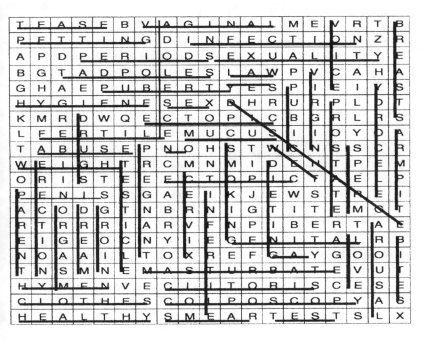

From June **1999** the prefix of many UK numbers alters. In London **0181 is replaced by 0208** and **0171 is replaced by 0207** - eg 0181 995 8782 will change to 0208 995 8782. **Freephone** numbers starting 0800 *may* change to a 0808 prefix instead. If in doubt please contact the operator. Every effort has been made to ensure that these numbers are correct at the time of publication.

HIV/AIDS
National AIDS helpline - free calls:
in English	0800 567 123
in Bengali, Gujerati, Hindi, Punjabi and Urdu	0800 371 134
in Cantonese	0800 282 446
in Arabic	0800 282 447
people hard of hearing	0800 521 361

National AIDS Trust   0207 972 2845
Scottish, Welsh, N Ireland & International AIDS helplines   0208 749 2828
Terrance Higgins Trust - HIV advice/ education   0207 242 1010
The NAZ Project - HIV/AIDS support to Asian, Latin American and African community   0171 741 1879

Sexuality
Acceptance - advice/counselling for parents of gay men and lesbians   01795 661 463
Albany Trust - support with sexual identity issues   0208 767 1827
Beaumont Society - support for transvestite and trans-sexual people   01582 412 220
Bisexual helpline:
London   0208 569 7500
Edinburgh   0131 557 3620
GLAD - Gay and Lesbian legal advice - 7-9.30pm Mon-Thurs   0207 837 5212
Lesbian and Gay Switchboard (open 24 hour) - support line   0207 837 7324
NRG - lesbian, bisexual and gay group for under 25s in south east London   0207 620 1819
Stonewall - lesbian and gay equality organisation   0207 336 8860

Family Planning/Reproductive Health
British Pregnancy Advisory Service (BPAS) - privately run charity offering Family Planning, Well Woman, assisted fertility, abortion advice etc.   08457 30 40 30

Birth Control Trust - advice, information and research   0207 278 7242
Brook Advisory - contraception/advice centres nationally for under 25s   0207 713 9000
Contraceptive Education Service (CES) - FPA Helpline - 9am-7pm   0207 837 4044
Family Planning Association (FPA – UK) helpline   0207 837 5432
Human Fertilisation & Embryology Assn infertility assistance   0207 377 5077
International Planned Parenthood Federation   0207 487 7900
Marie Stopes International - similar to PAS and BPAS   0207 388 4843
Marriage Care - Fertility UK - Roman Catholic organisation   0207 371 1341
Miscarriage Association   01924 200 799
National Association of NFP Teachers (Natural Family Planning)   0121 472 3806
Natural Childbirth Trust (NCT)   0208 992 8637
Pregnancy Advisory Service - similar to Marie Stopes above   0207 637 8962
Psychosexual Medicine – Institute of (they keep a register of Doctors who specialise in psycho-sexyal medicine)   0207 580 0631
Sex Education Forum - information source   0207 834 6025
Sexwise - confidential helpline for teenagers   0800 282 930

For people with disabilities
RNIB - Royal National Institute for the Blind   0345 023 153
RNID - Royal National Institute for the Deaf   0207 296 8000
SPOD - information/advice about sexual problems for the disabled   0207 607 8851
Outsiders Ltd - PO Box 4ZB, London W1A 4ZB - membership organisation - *'Always there for those who feel isolated or rejected.'* (no phone given)

Drugs
Alcoholics Anonymous   0207 352 3001
Cocaine Anonymous   0207 284 1123
CODA (Co-dependants Anonymous for dysfunctional families)   0207 376 8191
CITA - Council for Involuntary Tranquillizer Addiction   0151 949 0102
Families Anonymous - support for relatives or friends of people with drug problem   0207 498 4680

Mainliners Ltd - support for HIV and/or Hepatitis B/C positive people and injecting drug users
0207 582 5434

Narcotics Anonymous - support for relatives or friends of people with drug problem
0207 730 0009

National Drugs Helpline - advice and/or referral for help
0800 77 66 00

Network Scotland - information on drug related services in Scotland
0141 357 1774

SCODA (Standing Conference on Drug Addiction) - information on drug related services in England and Wales
0207 928 9500

Release - support on legal issues related to drugs and to families of users
0207 729 9904

Domestic/other violence and abuse

Childline - advice and support for children
0800 11 11

Childline - for children in care - lines open 5-10pm
0800 88 44 44

Consent - helps male survivors of sexual abuse and rape, their family and friends
0207 613 5486

Crimestoppers - free, confidential way to give Police information
0800 555 111

Everyman Centre - helps men with a history of violence
0207 737 6747

Survivors - offers support for people sexually abused by relatives
0208 833 3737

NSPCC (National Association for the Prevention of Cruelty to Children)
0800 800 800

Police - *CrimeStoppers*
0800 555 111

Police - in Emergency
999

Victim Support
0207 820 0007

Rape Crisis
0207 916 5466

Rape Crisis *counselling line*
0207 837 1600

Samaritans
0345 90 90 90

Women's Aid - out of London
0345 023 468

Women's Aid - London
0207 392 2092

General information

Alone in London - information for people under 21, single and homeless
0207 278 4224

Amarant Trust - menopause helpline
01293 413 000

Bacup - support for people with cancer
0207 267 1361

Blackliners - HIV and sexual health support to the Black community
0207 738 5274

Breast Care and Mastectomy Assn
0207 867 1103

British Liver Trust - advice/support for people concerned about hepatitis
0808 800 1000

Forward - support for women after circumcision, London
0171 725 2606

Forward Project - support for Black people with mental health problems aged 18-35
0207 381 8778

Health Education Authority
0207 413 1995

Health Education Board for Scotland
0131 536 5500

Health Information First - general health info. helpline
0800 66 55 44

Herpes Virus Association - supports people with/worried about herpes
0207 609 9061

National Council for One Parent Families
0207 267 1361

National Missing Persons Helpline
0500 700 700

National NEWPIN - support group for fathers/step fathers
0207 703 6326

Parentline
01702 559 900

Relate - couple and relationship counselling
01788 573 241

Refugee Council
0207 820 3000

Shelter – housing helpline
0808 800 4444

Women's Health (info)
0207 251 6580

Mail order condom, lubricant and other safer sex product retailers:

Condomania Ltd, Freepost RG3013, Thatcham, Berks RG19 4XA
01635 874 393
Website: http://condoms4u.com
E-mail: condomania.uk@virgin.net

FP Sales Ltd
01856 749 333

Further reading:

Men and Sex by Bernard Zilbergeld - for all male sexual problems/worries

The Pill by Prof. John Guillebaud

Contraception - Your Questions Answered - by Prof. John Guillebaud

The New Diary of a Teenage Health Freak and **The Diary of the other Health Freak** by Dr Aidan MacFarlane & Dr A McPherson

SEXplained... the Uncensored Guide to Sexual Health by Helen Knox provides information on sexually transmitted infections for *all* ages. See page 173 and the end of this book for more **SEXplained...**® information.

Contents & Index

Contents

Index

Knox Publishing
PO Box 6969
Chiswick
London W4 3WX – UK

Tel: 0207 995 8782 (0181 prior to June 99)
Web site: www.sexplained.com
E-mail: helen.knox@virgin.net

Mail order form for
SEXplained...® Books

Customer details   Please PRINT

Date: ....
Name: ....
Address: ....
....
....
Post code: .... Contact 'phone number: ....

Please send me .... copies of
SEXplained... The Uncensored Guide to Sexual Health
at £9.99 (sterling) plus £1.50 UK p&p (£3.00 overseas) (UK £11.49 each)
                     Price £ ....

Please send me .... copies of
SEXplained 2... For Young People
at £9.99 (sterling) plus £1.50 UK p&p (£3 overseas) (UK £11.49 each)
                     Price £ ....

Publisher's special offer:

Please send me copies of **The SEXplained...® Set** *(both books)*
at £15 plus £3.00 UK p&p (total £18.00)
or at £15 plus £5.00 overseas p&p (total £20)
                     Price £ ....

I enclose my cheque/postal order or Eurocheque made payable to **KNOX PUBLISHING**
to the sum of   £ ....

or

For credit card payment by **Mastercard, Visa or Eurocard**

Please debit my .... credit card account to the sum of £ ....
Card number ....
Card issue number ....
Card expiry date ....
Cardholder's address *(if different from above)* ....
....
Delivery address *(if different from above)* ....
....
Please state where you obtained or heard of **SEXplained...® Books**
....

Please allow 28 days for delivery   VAT No: 662 7730
Knox Publishing, PO Box 6969, Chiswick, London, W4 3WX, UK
Orders are also accepted if you write to KNOX PUBLISHING, with details and payment.

SEXplained...® © 1... Helen Knox

04357008